# INTEGRATIVE MEDICINE 2.0

*Thesis Doctor of Medicine in Alternative Medicine*

"In my view, the lost art of listening and ignoring the patient as a human being is a quintessential failure of our health care."

Copyright: Mirco Schieren (Herausgeber), 2017

Amazon Create Space

ISBN Paperback: 978-1545059128

Amazon Title-ID: 7054416

Thesis for Doctor of Medicine M.D. (AM), IBAM Kolkata, 80 Chowringhee Road, Kolkata 700020, India

Bibliografische Information der Deutschen Nationalbibliothek:

Die Deutsche Nationalbibliothek verzeichnet diese Publikation in der Deutschen Nationalbibliografie; detaillierte bibliografische Daten sind im Internet über http://dnb.d-nb.de abrufbar.

## Introduction

From my perspective it is important to understand, that integrative medicine – combining modern medicine and alternative medicine may lead us to a better future in health system. We can treat acute pain and diseases with modern medicine, ICUs and Stroke Units are high performance treatment entities – no doubt, but for example it is evident that convalescence is much more effectively when ICU rooms have windows with a view. What means that for integrative medicine? We need both systems. We need technical equipment, trained surgeons and specialists in acute situations, but in the same way we need treatments and approaches to support self-healing powers in convalescence.

Today a lot of patients and physicians are quite more open to discuss integrative medical treatment approaches, especially in pain management cases. In future we should try to work together in integrative teams to optimize treatment and medication standards and provide them to patients. More than 40 % of people in the US are using various forms of alternative medicines, 70 % of german primary care physicians prescribe one or more of nearly 700 phytomedicines (The Journal of Neuropsychiatry and Clinical Neurosciences 2000; 12:177-192). The literature reports that physician involvement is fairly low in the US; physician awareness of therapies has been shown to be only 19.7% for patients using complementary and conventional medicines and only 2.2% for patients using unconventional therapies. Patient disclosure to a physician also occurs at very low rates. One survey found that 63% of respondents did not disclose at least alternative therapy to their providers. The reasons for nondisclosure varied and included belief by the patient that it was unimportant, fear of physician disapproval, or active discouragement by the physician. Disclosure of CAM use by patients to their primary care providers becomes important when discussing the adverse effects of various modalities and potential interactions with conventional treatment. Many herbal products have been shown to have toxic effects and drug-drug interactions with conventional pharmaceuticals (in Journal of American Medical Association, 2004 Vol. 164). In all cases of pain we have to establish a better pain management system with cross boarder treatments and different therapy techniques.

A postoperative long time medication with opioid analgesics as single treatment is not an adequate pain management and can't be gold standard in the future. Along medical treatment mobilization, self-confidence training and social empowerment are highly recommended and evident for convalescence. So we need cross border treatment approaches, physician and health professional acceptance, better networking of therapists in the different fields of health. Hospitals could support this working-together-model with recommendations to its patients. In Germany primary care physicians tend to recommend and prescribe more and more alternative medical support. Psychotherapy and osteopathy are commonly insurance benefits from medical insurances in Germany. The following studies from the US will show the need for integration of alternative medicine and the willingness of health professionals to work together.

STUDY 1: Integration of complementary and alternative medicine in primary care: what do patients want? Jong MC, van de Vijver L, Busch M, Fritsma J, Seldenrijk R. (PubMed, U.S. National Library of Medicine 2012 Dec; 89(3):417-22. doi: 10.1016/j.pec.2012.08.013. Epub 2012 Sep 30)

To explore patients' perspectives towards integration of Complementary and Alternative Medicine (CAM) in primary care a mixed-methods approach was used. This included a survey on use, attitudes and disclosure of CAM, an e-panel consultation and focus group among patients with joint diseases. RESULTS: A total of 416 patients responded to the survey who suffered from osteoarthritis (51%), rheumatoid arthritis (29%) or fibromyalgia (24%). Prevalence of CAM use was 86%, of which 71% visited a CAM practitioner. Manual therapies, acupuncture and homeopathy were most frequently used. A minority (30%) actively communicated CAM use with their General Practitioner (GP). The majority (92%) preferred a GP who informed about CAM, 70% a GP who referred to CAM, and 42% wanted GPs to collaborate with CAM practitioners. Similar attitudes were found in the focus group and upon e-panel consultation.

The conclusion is that more patients in primary care want a GP who listens, inquire about CAM and if necessary refers to or collaborates with CAM practitioners.
PRACTICE IMPLICATIONS: To meet needs of patients, primary care disease management would benefit from an active involvement of GPs concerning CAM communication/referral. This study presents a model addressing the role of patients and GPs within such an integrative approach.

STUDY 2: Providing Complementary and Alternative Medicine in primary care: the primary care workers' perspective, van Haselen RA, Reiber U, Nickel I, Jakob A, Fisher PA (PubMed, U.S. National Library of Medicine, Complement Ther Med. 2004 Mar;12(1):6-16.)
The use of Complementary and Alternative Medicine (CAM) in primary care is growing, but still not widespread. Little is known about how CAM can/should be integrated into mainstream care.
To assess primary care health professionals' perceptions of need and of some ways to integrate CAM in primary care Questionnaire survey of primary health care workers in Northwest London. General Practitioners (GPs) were targeted in a postal survey, other members of the primary care team, such as district and practice nurses, were targeted via colleagues. The questionnaire assessed health care professionals' perspective on complementary medicine, referrals, ways to integrate complementary medicine into primary care and interest in research on CAM. RESULTS: Responses were obtained from 149 GPs (40% response rate after one reminder) and 24 nurses and 32 other primary care team members. One hundred and seventy-one (83%) respondents had previously referred (or influenced referral) for CAM treatments, the main reasons cited were: patients request (68%), conventional treatments failed (58%) and evidence (36%) (more than one reason could be given). Acupuncture and homoeopathy were the therapies for which patients were most frequently referred, followed by manual therapies. There was a significant interest in more training/information on CAM (66%). Only 12 respondents (6%) were against any integration of CAM in mainstream primary care. Most respondents felt that CAM therapies should be provided by doctors (66%) or other health professionals trained in CAM (82%). Twenty-six percent of respondents agreed with provision of CAM by non-state-registered practitioners. It was felt that the integration of CAM could lead to cost savings (70%), particularly in conditions involving pain, but also cost increases (55%) particularly in 'poorly defined conditions'. Fifty-six percent of respondents would consider participating in studies investigating CAM. The greatest interest was in acupuncture (41% of those who expressed an interest in research), homoeopathy (30%) and therapeutic massage/aromatherapy (26%).

There is considerable interest in CAM among primary care professionals, and many are already referring or suggesting referral. Such referrals are driven mainly by patient demand and by dissatisfaction with the results of conventional medicine. Most of the respondents were in favour of integrating at least some types of CAM in mainstream primary care. There is an urgent need to further educate and inform primary care health professionals about CAM and there is a broad need of clarifying work between physicians and patients to set up approaches for integrative medicine as working together model between traditional and alternative medicine. It is my fully belief, that a better world needs a better health system with physician's courage to humanity and a passionate understanding of what they do.

I declare that I have authored this paper independently as statutory declaration. It is important to say, that I am very thankful for support through my wonderful children and all the people around me day by day, thank you very much.

September 27, 2016
Mirco Schieren

## 1. *Principles and Philosophy of Alternative Medicine*

## Methods of Traditional Chinese Medicine (TCM)

a)        Moxibustion

Chinese medical treatment with burning "moxa wool" is to generate therapeutic heat on or near specific acupuncture points.  Moxibustion is a part of Chinese acupuncture and the pricking with needles, application of heat at local points at or near acupuncture points is to treat the yang deficiency states for yin diseases. It is induced in cases of chronic diseases like chronic bronchitis, chronic bronchial asthma, chronic diarrhea and arthritis where acupuncture or needling is forbidden or as an inadequate response.

b)        Oriental Diagnosis

Under this term we know the pulse diagnosis, known in the Traditional Chinese Medicine (TCM) and practiced in the oriental countries (f.eg. ayurvedic medicine system). In Ayurveda, advocates claim that by taking a pulse examination, humoral imbalances such as the three Doshas (Vata, Pitta, and Kapha) can be diagnosed. The ayurvedic pulse also claims to determine the balance of prana, tejas, and ojas. Ayurvedic pulse measurement is done by placing index, middle and ring finger on the wrist. The index finger is placed below the wrist bone on the thumb side of the hand (radial styloid). This finger represents the Vata dosha. The middle finger and ring finger are placed next to the index finger and represents consequently the Pitta and Kapha doshas of the patient. Pulse can be measured in the superficial, middle, and deep levels thus obtaining more information regarding energy imbalance of the patient.

In TCM the main sites for pulse assessment are the radial arteries in the left and right wrists, where it overlays the styloid process of the radius, between the wrist crease and extending proximal, approximately 5 cm in length. In traditional Chinese medicine, the pulse is divided into three positions on each wrist. The first pulse closest to the wrist is the cun position, the second guan, and the third pulse position furthest away from the wrist is the chi. There are several systems of diagnostic interpretation of pulse findings utilized in the Chinese medicine system. Some systems (Cun Kou) utilize overall pulse qualities, looking at changes in the assessed parameters of the pulse to derive one of the traditional 28 pulse types. Other approaches focus on individual pulse positions, looking at changes in the pulse quality and strength within the position, with each position having an association with a particular body area. For example, each of the paired pulse positions can represent the upper, middle and lower cavities of the torso, or are associated individually with specific organs. (For example, the small intestine is said to be reflected in the pulse at the left superficial position, and the heart at the deep position.) Various classic texts cite different arrangements to the pairings of organs, some omitting the second organ from the pulse entirely while others show organ systems reflecting the acupuncture channels (five phase pulse associations), and another the physical organ arrangement used in Chinese herbal medicine diagnosis (Li Shi Zhen). Generally, the commonly used organ associations are: first position on the left hand represents the heart and small intestine, the second, liver and gallbladder, and third the kidney yin and the bladder. On the right hand, the first position is representative of the lungs and large intestine, the second of the spleen and stomach, and the third represents the kidney yang and uterus or triple burner. The strengths and weaknesses of the positions are assessed at 3 depths each, namely fu (floating), zhong (middle) and chen (deep). These 9 positions are used to assess the patient diagnostically, along with the different qualities and speed of the pulse such as the Shu/Sun pulse classification system.

## Salient features and position of Alternative Medicine

Alternative medicines may be described as medical treatment systems outwards the mainstream of western medicine – practiced by a lot of physicians upcoming the last years, but with a long period of ignorance and misunderstanding in the western hemisphere.

Alternative medicine is as old as the oldest documentations may reach back, commonly part of the nature and the human nature to heal diseases. The understanding of the humans as part of the nature is important for each holistic approach of treatment and healing all kinds of diseases. There is not only one definition for alternative medicines – there may be a lot of definitions for each therapeutic method with spread all over the world. There may be no differences in performance and outcome inner each healing system. Each patient is different to another and it is important to know, that each method may be successful. The most salient features are as follows: 1. Health is defined as a state of physical wellbeing and it is important to know that the triad social, spiritual and physical (or body, mind and soul in Ayurveda) are important for that state of wellbeing. 2. There are more aspects and circumstances upon the maintenance of health, for example stress, proper diet, sexuality, positive attitudes, clean environment are promotive aspects of health. 3. The Simplicity of Treatment is important. Every treatment method has its own philosophy, diagnosis and treatments. 4. Less or no side effects 5. Alternative medicines give answers for nearly all kinds of diseases. Modern medical treatment is not able to answer important questions for diseases like psychosomatic disorders, degenerative disorders or diseases of bones and joints. 6. Fate – we can work with positive faith and positive faith is highly important for the development of self-healing power. We know that we can be successful where modern medicine is not even able to be. That sounds magic, but it simply follows the principles of nature.

## Definition of Aromatherapy

Aromatherapy offers diverse physical and psychological benefits, depending on the essential oil or oil combination and method of application used. Some common medicinal properties of essential oils used in aromatherapy include: analgesic, antimicrobial, antiseptic, anti-inflammatory, astringent, sedative, antispasmodic, expectorant, diuretic, and sedative. Essential oils are used to treat a wide range of symptoms and conditions, including, but not limited to, gastrointestinal discomfort, skin conditions, menstrual pain and irregularities, stress-related conditions, mood disorders, circulatory problems, respiratory infections, and wounds.

Aromatic plants have been employed for their healing, preservative, and pleasurable qualities throughout recorded history in both the East and West. As early as 1500 B.C. the ancient Egyptians used waters, oils, incense, resins, and ointments scented with botanicals for their religious ceremonies.

There is evidence that the Chinese may have recognized the benefits of herbal and aromatic remedies much earlier than this. The oldest known herbal text, Shen Nung's Pen Ts'ao (c. 2700-3000 B.C.) catalogs over 200 botanicals. Ayurveda, a practice of traditional Indian medicine that dates back over 2,500 years, also used aromatic herbs for treatment.

The Romans were well-known for their use of fragrances. They bathed with botanicals and integrated them into their state and religious rituals. So did the Greeks, with a growing awareness of the medicinal properties of herbs, as well. Greek physician and surgeon Pedanios Dioscorides, whose renown herbal text De Materia Medica (60 A.D.) was the standard textbook for Western medicine for 1,500 years, wrote extensively on the medicinal value of botanical aromatics. The Medica contained detailed information on over 500 plants and 4,740 separate medicinal uses for them, including an entire section on aromatics.

Written records of herbal distillation are found as early as the first century A.D., and around 1000 A.D., the noted Arab physician and naturalist Avicenna described the distillation of rose oil from rose petals, and the medicinal properties of essential oils in his writings. However, it wasn't until 1937, when French chemist René-Maurice Gattefossé published Aromatherapie: Les Huiles essentielles, hormones végé tales, that aromatherapie, or aromatherapy, was introduced in Europe as a medical discipline. Gattefossé, who was employed by a French perfumeur, discovered the healing properties of lavender oil quite by accident when he suffered a severe burn while working and used the closest available liquid, lavender oil, to soak it in.

In the late 20th century, French physician Jean Valnet used botanical aromatics as a front line treatment for wounded soldiers in World War II. He wrote about his use of essential oils and their healing and antiseptic properties, in his 1964 book Aromatherapie, traitement des maladies par les essences des plantes, which popularized the use of essential oils for medical and psychiatric treatment throughout France. Later, French biochemist Mauguerite Maury popularized the cosmetic benefits of essential oils, and in 1977 Robert Tisserand wrote the first English language book on the subject, The Art of Aromatherapy, which introduced massage as an adjunct treatment to aromatherapy and sparked its popularity in the United Kingdom.

In aromatherapy, essential oils are carefully selected for their medicinal properties. As essential oils are absorbed into the bloodstream through application to the skin or inhalation, their active components trigger certain pharmalogical effects (e.g., pain relief).

In addition to physical benefits, aromatherapy has strong psychological benefits. The volatility of an oil, or the speed at which it evaporates in open air, is thought to be linked to the specific psychological effect of an oil. As a rule of thumb, oils that evaporate quickly are considered emotionally uplifting, while slowly-evaporating oils are thought to have a calming effect.

## Complementary Medicine and how the subject helps in Integrated Medicine

To describe the complementary medicine with some words is not as simple as it seems to be. It came up for a long time ago in different cultures with different histories. Complementary medicine is defined by Eisenberg et al (in Journal of American Medical Association, 2004 Vol. 164) as "medical interventions not taught widely at medical schools or generally available at hospitals." These interventions are currently termed complementary and alternative medicines (CAMs). Complementary medicine and alternative medicine are not synonymous. Complementary medicine applies to nonallopathic treatment used in conjunction with standard medical care, whereas alternative medicine applies to treatment use in place of standard medical care. The National Institutes of Health groups CAM into the following 5 classes: alternative medicine practices, mind-body interventions, biologic-based therapies, manipulative and body-based methods, and energy modalities. Homeopathy, herbal supplements, massage, and chiropractic are various examples of these therapies.

Another definition for alternative medicine is the following: Alternative medicine is the term for medical products and practices that are not part of standard care. Standard care is what medical doctors, doctors of osteopathy, and allied health professionals, such as nurses and physical therapists, practice. Alternative medicine is used in place of standard medical care. An example is treating heart disease with chelation therapy (which seeks to remove excess metals from the blood) instead of using a standard approach. Examples of alternative practices include homeopathy, traditional medicine, chiropractic, and acupuncture. Complementary medicine is different from alternative medicine. Whereas complementary medicine is used together with conventional medicine, alternative medicine is used in place of conventional medicine. For the development of alternative medicines it is important, that we find coping strategies for all the peoples doubtfulness based upon misunderstandings, not given or wanting standards in alternative treatments and medication practice. We have to develop standards and requirements to bring up more credibility to complementary and alternative medicines. Furthermore physicians should be open to discuss allopathic or homeopathic treatment strategies to integrate this kind of alternative medicine in the health service.

## Manipulative Techniques

a) Physiotherapy is a manipulative technique and the deformities of a patient are modified in order to tonify the body and vital organs. It is practiced as a part of naturopathy. Physiotherapy helps the body to return back to life by natural principles and to bring back the harmony in mental, physical and spiritual fields, so that diseases can be prevented. The self-cleaning of a morbid individual by nature cure enhances the self-curative force of the body so that the body`s own defensive mechanisms are increased with purification of blood, proper distribution of nutrition throughout the body, proper functioning of all glands and organs with elimination of toxic and waste material from the body. Physiotherapy plays an important role for circulatory and muscular-neurological improvements and removal of wastes for the process of the bodies cleansing and regeneration.

Scientific exercises increase the functional ability of the organs and the body. Physiotherapy has wide curative effects as follows.

Assisting neuromuscular tension and toning up the nervous system, it helps to revitalize the vital force and enhance the immunity mechanisms, removes the accumulated body wastes, poisons, foreign substances and it helps the body in cleansing and regenerating by stimulation of glands and organs, it aids to regulate the blood vessels, lymphatics, muscles, tissues, tendons, bones, ligaments from all undue pressure, possible deformities and obstructions, to develop weak muscles, tendons, ligaments and other necessary adjustments, it improves coordination of movement, increases mobility of joints and defective postures. In sum we have to know, that physical medicine corrects all discoverable abnormalities of the body in all forms. Physiotherapy with its broad field of inducement and a long history back to first Egyptian manuscripts explaining scientific massage is one of the most popular naturopathic methods, often recommended through primary care physicians and as part of postoperative clinical treatments.

b) Chiropractic is a form of alternative medicine concerned with the diagnosis and treatment of mechanical disorders of the musculoskeletal system, especially the spine, under the belief that such a disorder affects general health via the nervous system. The main chiropractic treatment technique involves manual therapy, especially manipulation of the spine, other joints, and soft tissues, but may also include exercises and health and lifestyle counseling. The "specific focus of chiropractic practice" is chiropractic subluxation. Traditional chiropractic assumes that a vertebral subluxation or spinal joint dysfunction interferes with the body's function and its innate intelligence.

Chiropractic is well established in the United States, Canada, and Australia. It overlaps with other manual-therapy professions, including massage therapy, osteopathy, and physical therapy. Most who seek chiropractic care do so for low back pain, and back and neck pain are considered the specialties of chiropractic, but many chiropractors treat ailments other than musculoskeletal issues. Chiropractic has two main groups: "straights", now the minority emphasize vitalism, "innate intelligence" and spinal adjustments, and consider vertebral subluxations to be the cause of all disease; "mixers", the majority, are more open to mainstream views and conventional medical techniques, such as exercise, massage, and ice therapy. Many chiropractors describe themselves as primary care providers. D. D. Palmer founded chiropractic in the 1890s, and his son B. J. Palmer helped to expand it in the early 20th century. Throughout its history, chiropractic has been controversial. Its foundation is at odds with mainstream medicine, and has been sustained by pseudoscientific ideas such as subluxation and innate intelligence. The American Medical Association called chiropractic an "unscientific cult" in 1966 and boycotted it until losing an antitrust case in 1987. Chiropractic has had a strong political base and sustained demand for services; in recent decades, it has gained more legitimacy and greater acceptance among conventional physicians and health plans in the U.S., and evidence-based medicine has been used to review research studies and generate practice guidelines.

## Treatment of Alternative Medicines as holistic ones

The best way to understand the holistic approach in alternative medicine is a comparison. A comparison of alternative medicines with other forms of medicine (modern medicine f.eg.) is not even simple. But when we focus the most important differences we see, that the modern medicine is very diagnosis oriented. Making a diagnosis and a quick treatment, not even with a holistic view or approach is an enormous dilemma of modern medicine because we simply cannot adequately label so much of what we see and so we feel inadequate ourselves. The patient is not a car with an accident. He is more than an Ulcus Duodeni or a ruptured artery. What we see (symptoms) is only a part of a dysfunctional human system, but alternative medicines treats the body, mind and soul as a complex human system with self-healing power. Unfortunately all our ideas and concepts of life are restricted by our five physical senses and we try to understand all things based upon this. In order really to understand the complexity of our world, our life and our physical status or the pathogenesis of diseases we have to cast off our restrictive ways and envisage a real world larger than that which most of us appreciate with our five physical senses. In alternative medicines we know this and we know that the solely intellectual approach to science generally and medicine in particular is not providing the answers. The search for the perfect physician or the perfect medical mechanic, takes people from specialist to specialist in the hope of finding answers to chronic diseases that no one can explain, let alone cure. We in western society are greatly over doctored and interfered with and it is all of our own making.

It is important that the medical profession will have to come down from its pedestal and start accepting that it might not have all the answers. This will be the most difficult change to make because public faith and adulation over the years have built up doctors up to believe that they are much more able to cope with diseases than in fact they are. If we trust our knowledge, our senses and use empathy and try to treat a patient with a holistic approach – open to accept the opposite medical system and work side by side with medical professionals of the different systems, alternative and modern medicine – that's the way we can be even more successful with a kind of integrative medical treatment, with scope on a patient needs.

## The position of Alternative Medicines in India and abroad

In India alternative medicines is well accepted and courses of alternative medicines are offered by a lot of universities. The government of India has established a separate department for promotion of alternative medicines. A lot of NGOs are promoting alternative healing methods all over the country with good acceptance. In 1991 the High Court in Calcutta decided, that alternative medicine is allowed to practice without ban. In international contextual relation it is important to know that the World Health Organization WHO recognized and included these important practices in its program "Health for all by 2000 AD" and a lot of countries are following them with different projects and recommendations of and for using different kinds of alternative medical and accordingly low cost methods and treatments for everyone in the world.

## Biochemical medicines and its philosophy

The word 'Biochemistry' comes from the Greek 'Bios' for 'Life', coupled with 'Chemistry', the science that studies the composition of elements and the changes they go through. In the therapeutic sphere, Biochemistry is the system of treatment that uses the tissue remedies (inorganic salts of the body tissues) as medicine.

Dr. Wilhelm Heinrich Schuessler of Oldenburg, Germany, was a physician and a physiological chemist. He is credited with propagating the use of the twelve cell salts that are used in biochemistry, their practical use and the detailing of the Materia Medica on which this system is based. The earliest reference we can find to the use of the tissue remedies by Dr. Schuessler, is in an article that appeared in March 1873, titled "An Abridged Homoeopathic Therapeutics", the original in German, of course. The theory was refined with time, and was scrutinized and practiced by various respected physicians of the era, and found valuable in therapeutics. Over a period of time, Schuessler determined that Biochemistry was an independent branch of medicine, not to be absorbed into or related to homeopathy.

He insisted that its effects were by direct action, unlike homeopathy that worked probably by indirect Biochemic action. While there are those who practice biochemistry exclusively, and quite effectively, the consensus of opinion would probably suggest that it be used in conjunction with homeopathy. The methods of preparation of Biochemic and Homeopathic remedies are identical. Traditionally, Biochemic remedies are used in low potencies – 3x, 6x, 12x, up to 30x, while Homeopathic remedies are used in potencies varying from the low to the very high (CM, LM). Schuessler and orthodox Biochemic practitioners also insisted on the use of a single remedy, as in classical Homeopathy.

The difference in their use in the two systems is more a matter of theory. According to Dr. Schuessler, a deficiency of a certain cell salt gives rise to certain symptoms which point to its use as a remedy, and cure is affected by the restoration of the equilibrium of the salt in the body. The Homeopathic prescribing is done on the basis of 'Provings', and matches to patient symptoms the remedy that has been 'Proved' to cause those symptoms in a healthy person. It was always a question of debate as to how Homeopathic remedies effected cure. The correctly chosen remedy was presumed to tune the body's natural healing abilities – the 'Vital force' – to overcome disease. Dr. Schuessler claimed that Homeopathy worked indirectly through Biochemic principles, since very many Homeopathic remedies contain one or more of the tissue salts. The greater the proportion of a salt in a (homeopathic) remedy, the greater the resemblance between the two (e.g. Pulsatilla and Kali Sulph, which both have among their leading indications, aggravation in a warm room and in the evenings, and amelioration in the open air.) Both Aconite and Arnica contain Ferrum Phos and the similarities between the remedies are to be noted. Similarly there are many points of likeness between Hepar Sulph and Calc Sulph. Schuessler suggested that Biochemistry rectifies disease directly, by the administration of homogeneous substances, while Homeopathy does so indirectly, by the administration of heterogeneous substances. Biochemistry works on sound and valid principles. The two systems can be said to be siblings under the skin.

## Definition of Zone Therapy, Acupressure, Electrohomeopathy and Homeopathy

a) This ancient therapy can be traced to the Egyptians. It is the origin of hand and foot reflexology. The zones also have a relationship to the acupressure circuitry. Zone therapy is a simple therapy. Anyone can do it. With zone therapy, the body is divided by vertical lines into five zones on the left side and five zones on the right side. These zones relate to all parts of the body within each zone. The fingers and toes affect corresponding parts of the body and are the primary areas of treatment. Zone therapy works more directly on nerve endings that are connected with organs along the zones. This therapy is a very effective technique for pain release. Primary emphasis is on the hands and feet, with a focus being on the fingers and toes. These parts of the body have the least depth to them. Nerve endings in these areas are near the surface and thus more accessible. The procedure is to press down using a circular, rolling motion. Look for the tender spots, using a constant kind of pressure.

If no tenderness is found, gently and slowly pressing deeper until the tenderness is found. Key on sensitivity. Apply pressure on the upper and lower surfaces as well as the sides of the fingers and toes. Do one area at a time, massaging all tender spots. When starting, pinpoint massage an area only for a few seconds, then let the area rest while you massage another spot. Keep coming back for a few seconds each time until the sensitivity is gone. Do not over-massage at the beginning; proceed slowly. Stimulate each tender spot at first for a maximum of 30 seconds. Increase pressure when tolerance has been established. Be persistent. For maximum effect, apply pressure for 30 seconds to four minutes, depending on the severity of the tenderness. Any tenderness is an indication of some degree of congestion in the associated zone. There is little written information on Zone Therapy. This is an opportunity to experiment, using your sensitivity and intuition.

Pinching the thumb and index finger together are the best instruments for fine in-depth stimulation. Pressure may also be applied with a blunt point applicator like a pencil with a rubber eraser. Clothespins may be used to apply strong, steady pressure. Pocket combs can be used along a wide area, clenching the fist to press the teeth of the comb against the inner surfaces of the fingers.

When massaging, cover all possible zones for a specific organ. Strong pressure on the tip of the thumb or big toe affects the whole first zone. Similar pressure on the tips of the other fingers and toes will affect corresponding zones. For example, an organ like the liver lies in all five zones on the right side and the eyes correspond with the three middle fingers and toes. The eyes relate to zones 3, 4, and 5. Pain anywhere in a particular zone will be lessened through pressure on the corresponding finger and toe. Pressure applied on the outside of the fingers and toes will be felt on the front of the body. Pressure on the inside of the fingers and the bottom of the toes will be expressed in the back.

b) Electrohomoeopathy (or Mattei cancer cure) is a derivative of homeopathy invented in the 19th century by Count Cesare Mattei. The name is derived from a combination of electro (referring to an electric bio-energy content supposedly extracted from plants and of therapeutic value, rather than electricity in its conventional sense) and homeopathy (referring to an alternative medicinal philosophy developed by Samuel Hahnemann in the 18th century). Electrohomeopathy has been defined as the combination of electrical devices and homeopathy.

Remedies are derived from what are said to be the active micro nutrients or mineral salts of certain plants. One contemporary account of the process of producing electrohomeopathic remedies was as follows:

As to the nature of his remedies we learn ... that ... they are manufactured from certain herbs, and that the directions for the preparation of the necessary dilutions are given in the ordinary jargon of homeopathy. The globules and liquids, however, are "instinct with a potent, vital, electrical force, which enables them to work wonders". This process of "fixing the electrical principle" is carried on in the secret central chamber of a Neo-Moorish castle which Count Mattei has built for himself in the Bolognese Apennines ... The "red electricity" and "white electricity" supposed to be "fixed" in these "vegetable compounds" are in their very nomenclature and suggestion poor and miserable fictions. According to Mattei's own ideas however, every disease originates in the change of blood or of the lymphatic system or both, and remedies can therefore be mainly divided into two broad categories to be used in response to the dominant affected system. Mattei wrote that having obtained plant extracts, he was "able to determine in the liquid vegetable electricity". Allied to his theories and therapies were elements of Chinese medicine, of medical humours, of apparent Brownianism, as well as modified versions of Samuel Hahnemann's homeopathic principles. Electrohomeopathy has some associations with Spagyric medicine, a holistic medical philosophy claimed to be the practical application of alchemy in medical treatment, so that the principle of modern electrohomeopathy is that disease is typically multi-organic in cause or effect and therefore requires holistic treatment that is at once both complex and natural.

A symposium took place in Bologna in 2008 to mark the 200th anniversary of the birth of Cesare Mattei, with attendees from India, Pakistan, Germany, UK, and the USA. Electrohomeopathy is practised predominantly in India and Pakistan (RAJYA SABHA Parliamentary Bulletin- The Recognition of Electro Homoeopathy System of Medicine Bill, 2015 by Dr. E. M. Sudarsana Natchiappan, M. P), but there are also a number of electrohomeopathy organizations and institutions worldwide.

## Zone Therapy and its detailed modus operandi in cure

Zone Therapy aka Reflexology is a therapeutic method of relieving pain by stimulating predefined pressure points on the feet and hands. This controlled pressure alleviates the source of the discomfort. In the absence of any particular malady or abnormality, reflexology may be as effective for promoting good health and for preventing illness as it may be for relieving symptoms of stress, injury, and illness. Reflexologists work from maps of predefined pressure points that are located on the hands and feet. These pressure points are reputed to connect directly through the nervous system and affect the bodily organs and glands. The reflexologist manipulates the pressure points according to specific techniques of reflexology therapy. By means of this touching therapy, any part of the body that is the source of pain, illness, or potential debility can be strengthened through the application of pressure at the respective foot or hand location.

Reflexology promotes healing by stimulating the nerves in the body and encouraging the flow of blood. In the process, reflexology not only quells the sensation of pain, but relieves the source of the pain as well. Anecdotally, reflexologists claim success in the treatment of a variety of conditions and injuries. One condition is fibromyalgia. People with this disease are encouraged to undergo reflexology therapy to alleviate any of a number of chronic bowel syndromes associated with the condition. Frequent brief sessions of reflexology therapy are also recommended as an alternative to drug therapy for controlling the muscle pain associated with fibromyalgia and for relieving difficult breathing caused by tightness in the muscles of the patient's neck and throat.

Reflexology applied properly can alleviate allergy symptoms, as well as stress, back pain, and chronic fatigue. The techniques of reflexology can be performed conveniently on the hand in situations where a session on the feet is not practical, although the effectiveness of limited hand therapy is less pronounced than with the foot pressure therapy. Reflexology is a healing art of ancient origin. Although its origins are not well documented, there are reliefs on the walls of a Sixth Dynasty Egyptian tomb (c. 2450 B.C.) that depict two seated men receiving massage on their hands and feet. From Egypt, the practice may have entered the Western world during the conquests of the Roman Empire. The concepts of reflexology have also been traced to pre-dynastic China (possibly as early as 3000 B.C.) and to ancient Indian medicine. The Inca civilization may have subscribed to the theories of reflexology and passed on the practice of this treatment to the Native Americans in the territories that eventually entered the United States. In recent times, Sir Henry Head first investigated the concepts underlying reflexology in England in the 1890s. Therapists in Germany and Russia were researching similar notions at approximately the same time, although with a different focus. Less than two decades later, a physician named William H. Fitzgerald presented a similar concept that he called zone analgesia or zone therapy. Fitzgerald's zone analgesia was a method of relieving pain through the application of pressure to specific locations throughout the entire body. Fitzgerald divided the body into 10 vertical zones, five on each side that extended from the head to the fingertips and toes, and from front toback. Every aspect of the human body appears in one of these 10 zones, and each zone has a reflex area on the hands and feet. Fitzgerald and his colleague, Dr. Edwin Bowers, demonstrated that by applying pressure on one area of the body, they could anesthetize or reduce pain in a corresponding part. In 1917, Fitzgerald and Bowers published Relieving Pain at Home, an explanation of zone therapy.

Later, in the 1930s, a physical therapist, Eunice D. Ingham, explored the direction of the therapy and made the startling discovery that pressure points on the human foot were situated in a mirror image of the corresponding organs of the body with which the respective pressure points were associated. Ingham documented her findings, which formed the basis of reflexology, in Stories the Feet Can Tell, published in 1938. Although Ingham's work in reflexology was inaccurately described as zone therapy by some, there are differences between the two therapies of pressure analgesia. Among the more marked differences, reflexology defines a precise correlation between pressure points and afflicted areas of the body. Furthermore, Ingham divided each foot and hand into 12 respective pressure zones, in contrast to the 10 vertical divisions that encompass the entire body in Fitzgerald's zone therapy.

In 1968 two siblings, Dwight Byers and Eusebia Messenger, established the National Institute of Reflexology. By the early 1970s the institute had grown and was renamed the International Institute of Reflexology. In a typical reflexology treatment, the therapist and patient have a preliminary discussion prior to therapy, to enable the therapist to focus more accurately on the patient's specific complaints and to determine the appropriate pressure points for treatment. A reflexology session involves pressure treatment that is most commonly administered in foot therapy sessions of approximately 40-45 minutes in duration. The foot therapy may be followed by a brief 15-minute hand therapy session. No artificial devices or special equipment are associated with this therapy. The human hand is the primary tool used in reflexology. The therapist applies controlled pressure with the thumb and forefinger, generally working toward the heel of the foot or the outer palm of the hand. Most reflexologists apply pressure with their thumbs bent; however, some also use simple implements, such as the eraser end of a pencil. Reflexology therapy is not massage, and it is not a substitute for medical treatment. Reflexology is a complex system that identifies and addresses the mass of 7,000 nerve endings that are contained in the foot. Additional reflexology addresses the nerves that are located in the hand. This is a completely natural therapy that affords relief without the use of drugs. The Reflexology Association of America (RAA) formally discourages the use of oils or other preparations in performing this hands-on therapy.

In order to realize maximum benefit from a reflexology session, the therapist as well as the patient should be situated so as to afford optimal comfort for both. Patients in general receive treatment in a reclining position, with the therapist positioned as necessary—to work on the bare feet, or alternately on the bare hands. A reflexology patient removes both shoes and socks in order to receive treatment. No other preparation is involved. No prescription drugs, creams, oils, or lotions are used on the skin. Reflexology is extremely safe. It may even be self-administered in a limited form whenever desired. The qualified reflexologist offers a clear and open disclaimer that reflexology does not constitute medical treatment in any form, nor is reflexology given as a substitute for medical advice or treatment. The ultimate purpose of the therapy is to promote wellness; fundamentally it is a form of preventive therapy.

## Various aspects of Alternative Medicines

In modern world we use modern medicine to treat diseases under different circumstances, like human resources of medical staff, time per treatment and costs of treatment and medication in the western hemisphere. In third world countries we have nearly the same problems but with much more problems to finance treatments, personal, technical and medical equipment. Based upon skills like cost limitation and cost reduction in the public sector and last but not least the effectiveness of treatments we have to compare the alternative medicines and modern medicine. Modern treatments commonly are focused on healing diseases not with a holistic view and approach under involvement of self-healing powers. In modern medicine, invasive methods and surgery are commonly used but not only to treat acute ailments and diseases. Surgical methods are also used to treat chronic diseases and pain symptoms. We know that modern medicine is high ranked and needed in acute life-threatening situations like cardiac, pulmonary and respiratory ailments, bone fractures and cartilage damages with famous performances. In chronic diseases and pain management we found out, that nearly 70 percent of surgical interventions are not as successful as needed to accept responsibility for. Bernard Lown, the inventor of the current defibrillator and a famous cardiologist stipulated more than 50 % of the patients with heart bypass interventions had significant brain injuries after these interventions. We know today, that a lot of these bypass interventions were obsolete in case of Nitroglycerine medication (from "A Maverick's Lonely Path in Cardiology", Bernard Lown, MD). Physicians commonly recommend patients bed rest and movement limitations. We know that these movement limitations bring patients to pain symptoms. Surgical treatments are high cost interventions with even partly limited success and high mortality rates up to 5%.

Non-invasive interventions are much more successful in pain management than surgical interventions. Analgesic medications have a lot of side effects and bring patients to substance abuse problems. In average 2 percent of the world population shows a medicine dependency in a wide range of opioid and non-opioid medications and not even analgesics. We know that homeopathic medications have limited or no side effects and there are a lot of controlled randomized clinical blind studies to verify the effectiveness of homeopathic medics. Osteopathy, Chiropractic or Hypnosis and support in developing a daily routine to manage and prevent from pain symptoms are sensitive methods with performance rates of about 70 percent in average. All of these alternative treatments are low cost labelled and no more cost intensive technical equipment is needed. Based upon foresaid alternative methods are fully qualified for practicing in poor or third world countries.

## 2. *Psychotherapy and Counselling*

### Definition of Psychotherapy and the types of Psychotherapy

Psychotherapy, or "talk therapy", is a way to treat people with a mental disorder by helping them understand their illness. It teaches people strategies and gives them tools to deal with stress and unhealthy thoughts and behaviours. Psychotherapy helps patients manage their symptoms better and function at their best in everyday life. Sometimes psychotherapy alone may be the best treatment for a person, depending on the illness and its severity. Other times, psychotherapy is combined with medications. Therapists work with an individual or families to devise an appropriate treatment plan.

Cognitive behavioural therapy (CBT) is a blend of two therapies: cognitive therapy (CT) and behavioural therapy. CT was developed by psychotherapist Aaron Beck, M.D., in the 1960's. CT focuses on a person's thoughts and beliefs, and how they influence a person's mood and actions, and aims to change a person's thinking to be more adaptive and healthy. Behavioural therapy focuses on a person's actions and aims to change unhealthy behaviour patterns.
Dialectical Behaviour Therapy

Dialectical behaviour therapy (DBT), a form of CBT, was developed by Marsha Linehan, Ph.D. At first, it was developed to treat people with suicidal thoughts and actions. It is now also used to treat people with borderline personality disorder (BPD). BPD is an illness in which suicidal thinking and actions are more common. The term "dialectical" refers to a philosophic exercise in which two opposing views are discussed until a logical blending or balance of the two extremes—the middle way—is found. In keeping with that philosophy, the therapist assures the patient that the patient's behaviour and feelings are valid and understandable. At the same time, the therapist coaches the patient to understand that it is his or her personal responsibility to change unhealthy or disruptive behaviour. DBT emphasizes the value of a strong and equal relationship between patient and therapist. The therapist consistently reminds the patient when his or her behaviour is unhealthy or disruptive—when boundaries are overstepped—and then teaches the skills needed to better deal with future similar situations. DBT involves both individual and group therapy. Individual sessions are used to teach new skills, while group sessions provide the opportunity to practice these skills. Research suggests that DBT is an effective treatment for people with BPD. A recent NIMH-funded study found that DBT reduced suicide attempts by half compared to other types of treatment for patients with BPD. CBT helps a person focus on his or her current problems and how to solve them. Both patient and therapist need to be actively involved in this process. The therapist helps the patient learn how to identify distorted or unhelpful thinking patterns, recognize and change inaccurate beliefs, relate to others in more positive ways, and change behaviours accordingly. CBT can be applied and adapted to treat many specific mental disorders.

Interpersonal Therapy (IPT) is most often used on a one-on-one basis to treat depression or dysthymia (a more persistent but less severe form of depression). The current manual-based form of IPT used today was developed in the 1980's by Gerald Klerman, M.D., and Myrna Weissman, M.D.

IPT is based on the idea that improving communication patterns and the ways people relate to others will effectively treat depression. IPT helps identify how a person interacts with other people. When a behaviour is causing problems, IPT guides the person to change the behaviour. IPT explores major issues that may add to a person's depression, such as grief, or times of upheaval or transition. Sometimes IPT is used along with antidepressant medications. IPT varies depending on the needs of the patient and the relationship between the therapist and patient. Basically, a therapist using IPT helps the patient identify troubling emotions and their triggers. The therapist helps the patient learn to express appropriate emotions in a healthy way. The patient may also examine relationships in his or her past that may have been affected by distorted mood and behaviour. Doing so can help the patient learn to be more objective about current relationship.

Family-focused therapy (FFT) was developed by David Miklowitz, Ph.D., and Michael Goldstein, Ph.D., for treating bipolar disorder. It was designed with the assumption that a patient's relationship with his or her family is vital to the success of managing the illness. FFT includes family members in therapy sessions to improve family relationships, which may support better treatment results. Therapists trained in FFT work to identify difficulties and conflicts among family members that may be worsening the patient's illness. Therapy is meant to help members find more effective ways to resolve those difficulties. The therapist educates family members about their loved one's disorder, its symptoms and course, and how to help their relative manage it more effectively. When families learn about the disorder, they may be able to spot early signs of a relapse and create an action plan that involves all family members. During therapy, the therapist will help family members recognize when they express unhelpful criticism or hostility toward their relative with bipolar disorder. The therapist will teach family members how to communicate negative emotions in a better way. Several studies have found FFT to be effective in helping a patient become stabilized and preventing relapses. FFT also focuses on the stress family members feel when they care for a relative with bipolar disorder. The therapy aims to prevent family members from "burning out" or disengaging from the effort. The therapist helps the family accept how bipolar disorder can limit their relative. At the same time, the therapist holds the patient responsible for his or her own well-being and actions to a level that is appropriate for the person's age.

Generally, the family and patient attend sessions together. The needs of each patient and family are different, and those needs determine the exact course of treatment.

Psychodynamic Therapy. Historically, psychodynamic therapy was tied to the principles of psychoanalytic theory, which asserts that a person's behaviour is affected by his or her unconscious mind and past experiences. Now therapists who use psychodynamic therapy rarely include psychoanalytic methods. Rather, psychodynamic therapy helps people gain greater self-awareness and understanding about their own actions. It helps patients identify and explore how their nonconscious emotions and motivations can influence their behaviour. Sometimes ideas from psychodynamic therapy are interwoven with other types of therapy, like CBT or IPT, to treat various types of mental disorders. Research on psychodynamic therapy is mixed. However, a review of 23 clinical trials involving psychodynamic therapy found it to be as effective as other established psychotherapies.

Play Therapy. This therapy is used with children. It involves the use of toys and games to help a child identify and talk about his or her feelings, as well as establish communication with a therapist. A therapist can sometimes better understand a child's problems by watching how he or she plays. Research in play therapy is minimal.

## The features of Mental Disorders

Mental health disorders occur in a variety of forms, and symptoms can overlap, making disorders hard to diagnoses. However, there are some common disorders that affect people of all ages.

*Attention Deficit Hyperactivity Disorder (ADHD)*
Attention Deficit Hyperactivity Disorder is characterized by an inability to remain focused on task, impulsive behaviour, and excessive activity or an inability to sit still. Although this disorder is most commonly diagnosed in children, it can occur in adults as well.

*Bipolar Disorder*

Bipolar disorder causes a periodic cycling of emotional states between manic and depressive phases. Manic phases contain periods of extreme activity and heightened emotions, whereas depressive phases are characterized by lethargy and sadness. The cycles do not tend to occur instantly.

*Depression*

Depression covers a wide range of conditions, typically defined by a persistent bad mood and lack of interest in pursuing daily life, as well as bouts of lethargy and fatigue. Dysthymia is a milder but longer-lasting form of depression.

*Schizophrenia*

Schizophrenia is not, as commonly thought, solely about hearing voices or having multiple personalities. Instead, it is defined by a lack of ability to distinguish reality. Schizophrenia can cause paranoia and belief in elaborate conspiracies. There is no single cause for mental health disorders; instead, they can be caused by a mixture of biological, psychological and environmental factors. People who have a family history of mental health disorders may be more prone to developing one at some point. Changes in brain chemistry from substance abuse or changes in diet can also cause mental disorders. Psychological factors and environmental factors such as upbringing and social exposure can form the foundations for harmful thought patterns associated with mental disorders. Mental health disorders exist in broad categories: anxiety disorders, mood disorders, psychotic disorders, personality disorders and impulse control disorders. If someone you know experiences erratic thought patterns, unexplained changes in mood, lack of interest in socializing, lack of empathy, inability to tell the difference between reality and fantasy, or a seeming lack of control, that person may have a mental health disorder. This is, by no means, a complete list of symptoms. Mental health problems can cause a wide variety of emotional symptoms, some of which include:

- *Changes in mood*
- *Erratic thinking*
- *Chronic anxiety*
- *Exaggerated sense of self-worth*
- *Impulsive actions*

Mental health problems typically do not cause physical symptoms in and of themselves. Depression, however, can indirectly cause weight loss, fatigue and loss of libido, among others. Eating disorders, a separate class of mental health disorders, can cause malnutrition, weight loss, amenorrhea in women, or electrolyte imbalances caused by self-induced vomiting. This makes eating disorders among the most deadly of mental health disorders. In the short-term, mental health problems can cause people to be alienated from their peers because of perceived unattractive personality traits or behaviours. They can also cause anger, fear, sadness and feelings of helplessness if the person does not know or understand what is happening. In the long-term, mental health disorders can drive a person to commit suicide. According to the National Institute for Mental Health, over 90 percent of suicides have depression or another mental disorder as factors.

## Definition of psychological practices and the Therapeutic Community Treatment Model

Practicing psychologists help a wide variety of people and can treat many kinds of problems. Some people may talk to a psychologist because they have felt depressed, angry or anxious for a long time. Or, they want help for a chronic condition that is interfering with their lives or physical health. Others may have short-term problems they want help navigating, such as feeling overwhelmed by a new job or grieving the death of a family member. Psychologists can help people learn to cope with stressful situations, overcome addictions, manage their chronic illnesses and break past the barriers that keep them from reaching their goals.

Practicing psychologists are also trained to administer and interpret a number of tests and assessments that can help diagnose a condition or tell more about the way a person thinks, feels and behaves. These tests may evaluate intellectual skills, cognitive strengths and weaknesses, vocational aptitude and preference, personality characteristics and neuropsychological functioning. Practicing psychologists can help with a range of health problems and use an assortment of evidence-based treatments to help people improve their lives. Most commonly, they use therapy (often referred to as psychotherapy or talk therapy). There are many different styles of therapy, but the psychologist will choose the type that best addresses the person's problem and best fits the patient's characteristics and preferences.

Some common types of therapy are cognitive, behavioural, cognitive-behavioural, interpersonal, humanistic, psychodynamic or a combination of a few therapy styles. Therapy can be for an individual, couples, family or other group. Some psychologists are trained to use hypnosis, which research has found to be effective for a wide range of conditions including pain, anxiety and mood disorders.

For some conditions, therapy and medication are a treatment combination that works best. For people who benefit from medication, psychologists work with primary care physicians, pediatricians and psychiatrists on their overall treatment.

Therapeutic communities (TCs) are a common form of long-term residential treatment for substance use disorders (SUDs). Residential treatment for SUDs emerged in the late 1950s out of the self-help recovery movement, which included groups such as Alcoholics Anonymous. Some such groups evolved into self-supporting and democratically run residences to support abstinence and recovery from drug use (Sacks & Sacks, 2010). Examples have included community lodges, Oxford Houses, and TCs. The first TC was the Synanon residential rehabilitation community, founded in 1958 in California. During the 1960s, the first generation of TCs spread throughout areas of the United States, and today the TC approach (see "What is a Therapeutic Community's Approach?") has been adopted in more than 65 countries around the world (Bunt et al., 2008).

Historically, TCs have seen themselves as a mutual self-help alternative to medically oriented strategies to address addiction and most have not allowed program participants to use medications of any kind, including medications such as methadone (a long-acting opioid agonist medication shown to be effective in treating opioid addiction and pain) (De Leon, 2000; De Leon, 2015). Over the past 30 years, TCs' attitudes toward medications have gradually evolved, reflecting changing social attitudes toward addiction treatment and the scientific recognition of addiction as a medical disorder (De Leon, 2000; De Leon, 2015; Vanderplasschen et al., 2013). A growing number of TCs now take a comprehensive approach to recovery by addressing participants' other health issues in addition to their SUDs, incorporating comprehensive medical treatment (Smith, 2012) and supporting participants receiving medications for addiction treatment or for other psychiatric disorders (see "How Are Therapeutic Communities Adapting to the Current Environment?"). Many of today's TCs are also offering shorter-term residential or outpatient day treatment (De Leon, 2012; De Leon & Wexler, 2009) in addition to long-term residential treatment.

TCs have also been adapted over time to address the treatment needs of different populations. During the 1990s, modified TCs emerged to treat people with co-occurring psychiatric disorders, homeless individuals, women, and adolescents (De Leon, 2010; Sacks et al., 2004b; Sacks et al., 2003; Sacks & Sacks, 2010; Jainchill et al., 2005) (see "How Do Therapeutic Communities Treat Populations with Special Needs?"). Also, as the proportion of offenders with SUDs rose during the same period, correctional institutions began incorporating in-prison TCs (often in separate housing units), and TCs are available for people re-entering society after prison with the goal of reducing both drug use and recidivism (Wexler & Prendergast, 2010) (see "How Are Therapeutic Communities Integrated into the Criminal Justice System?").

Initially, TCs were run solely by peers in recovery. Over time and in response to the changing needs of participants, many TCs have begun incorporating professional staff with substance abuse counselling or mental health training, some of whom are also in recovery themselves. Today, programs often have medically trained professionals (e.g., psychiatrist consultants, nurses, and methadone specialists) as staff members, and most offer medical services on-site.

## Definition of Counselling and the treatment of Traumatic Stress Disorders

Counselling is an interactive client beneficial relationship set up to approach a client's issues. These issues can be social, cultural and or emotional and the Counsellor will approach them in a holistic way. A client can be a person, or a family group or even an institution.

The overall aim of counselling is to help clients recognise opportunities to help them live in more satisfying and rewarding ways as individuals and as members of society. The Counsellor can be involved in resolving specific problems which could involve making decisions and helping a client cope when in a crisis situation. The Counsellor can help a client resolve relationship issues, through helping them raise their self-awareness. To do this they will also need to work with the client's feelings, thoughts and perceptions and be aware of both internal and external conflicts. It means the method that counsellors uses when they set aside time with a client to enable them together to discover a client's stressful or emotional feelings.

The method sets out to help the client to see things if possible from a different viewpoint perhaps see things more clearly. The purpose is to help the client to focus on their feelings or behaviour to bring about a positive change. It is a paramount importance that the counsellor helps to set up a relationship of trust where the client has explained to them the confidentiality of their meetings. It may be necessary to explain to the client that if they believe there is a risk to life they may be required by law to disclose information to perhaps their supervisor or a member of law enforcement.

Post-traumatic stress disorder (PTSD) was first used as a diagnosis by veterans from the Vietnam War, but such symptoms have existed for much longer. The disorder has had many names, including:

- *battle fatigue*
- *combat stress*
- *shell shock*
- *post-traumatic stress syndrome (PTSS)*

Post-traumatic stress disorder isn't only associated with war-related scenarios however. -Traumatic events such as natural disasters, abuse and accidents can also cause symptoms. It is understandable for people to feel distressed and upset after a traumatic event. For many, these feelings gradually subside and they are able to carry on with their lives as normal. For others however, distress and anxiety following a trauma may be ongoing. It can be so severe that their everyday lives and ability to live normally suffer.

Post-traumatic stress disorder develops after experiencing, or witnessing, a traumatic event. Typically, people in danger feel afraid. When this fear hits, the 'fight or flight' response is triggered. But for people with PTSD, this type of reaction is damaged. They may feel frightened or stressed even if they are no longer in danger. The threat of physical harm, or physical harm itself can cause post-traumatic stress disorder. To develop the condition, you could be:

- *the person who was harmed*
- *a close relation of the person that was harmed*
- *someone who witnessed a traumatic event that affected others*

You may even develop the disorder years after the event - there isn't a time limit on distress.If you have PTSD, you may relive the traumatic event through flashbacks and nightmares. You also may feel isolated, guilty and sometimes irritable. Sleeping problems such as insomnia are also common. Post-traumatic stress disorder symptoms are persistent and severe enough to impact your daily life.

As post-traumatic stress disorder is so complex, many who have it live their life undiagnosed, missing out on treatment. Some may feel uncomfortable talking about their feelings with others and do not want to admit they are struggling to cope after the trauma. There might be a fear of being perceived as emotionally unstable, or even weak. If this is so, their loved ones are usually kept in the dark in such matters.

If you are diagnosed with post-traumatic stress disorder you will be given access to specialised PTSD treatment. Such treatment including counselling for PTSD, can offer a private and confidential space to talk about your symptoms and feelings surrounding the trauma and condition. Counselling for PTSD aims to address issues that deeply affect people both physically and emotionally. Talking therapies are also effective in treating associated mental health conditions. These include anxiety, phobias and depression.

There are a number of approaches that can be used in counselling for PTSD. These include:

CBT for PTSD is where a therapist helps a client to understand their current thought patterns. This is so they can identify those that are harmful and unhelpful. Through this process, sufferers can come to terms with their trauma and gain a sense of control over their fear. By focusing on realistic thoughts, they can avoid falling back into negative thinking patterns whenever they encounter a trigger.

Eye movement desensitisation and reprocessing (EMDR), this approach aims to reduce symptoms of post-traumatic stress disorder via a series of side-to-side eye movements. EMDR addresses the brain differences in sufferers. It helps them to process memories and flashbacks of a trauma more effectively.

The human givens approach to psychotherapy lends itself well to the treatment of PTSD. The premise is based on how humans have a set of needs, or givens. If any of these givens are not met, it can cause psychological distress. The technique that human givens therapists tend to use is called 'the rewind technique'. This uses cognitive restructuring and imaginary exposure to remove the association between the memory of the trauma and the emotional response.

Counselling for complex PTSD

There is limited research into the treatment of complex PTSD. Yet, the methods and processes involved tend to be similar to the ones used in counselling for PTSD. Self-discovery and exploration of the trauma is a key part of treatment. This helps sufferers to come to terms with what has happened, accept that it was undeserved and find ways to overcome it. Recovery involves focusing on the problems that can be resolved to help sufferers to regain a sense of control.


## The concept and therapeutic utilities of psychological therapies

Psychotherapy is the use of psychological methods, particularly when based on regular personal interaction, to help a person change and overcome problems in desired ways. Psychotherapy aims to improve an individual's well-being and mental health, to resolve or mitigate troublesome behaviours, beliefs, compulsions, thoughts, or emotions, and to improve relationships and social skills. Certain psychotherapies are considered evidence-based for treating some diagnosed mental disorders. There are over a thousand different psychotherapies, some being minor variations, while others are based on very different conceptions of psychology, ethics (how to live) or techniques. Most involve one-to-one sessions, between client and therapist, but some are conducted with groups, including families.

Psychotherapists may be mental health professionals such as psychiatrists or psychologists, or come from a variety of other backgrounds, and depending on the jurisdiction may be legally regulated, voluntarily regulated or unregulated (and the term itself may be protected or not). The term psychotherapy is derived from Ancient Greek psyche (ψυχή meaning "breath; spirit; soul") and therapeia (θεραπεία "healing; medical treatment"). The Oxford English Dictionary defines it now as "The treatment of disorders of the mind or personality by psychological methods..."

The American Psychological Association adopted a resolution on the effectiveness of psychotherapy in 2012 based on a definition developed by John C. Norcross: "Psychotherapy is the informed and intentional application of clinical methods and interpersonal stances derived from established psychological principles for the purpose of assisting people to modify their behaviours, cognitions, emotions, and/or other personal characteristics in directions that the participants deem desirable". Influential editions of a work by psychiatrist Jerome Frank defined psychotherapy as a healing relationship using socially authorized methods in a series of contacts primarily involving words, acts and rituals—regarded as forms of persuasion and rhetoric.

Some definitions of counselling overlap with psychotherapy (particularly non-directive client-centered approaches), or counselling may refer to guidance for everyday problems in specific areas, typically for shorter durations with a less medical focus. Somatotherapy refers to the use of physical methods as treatments, and sociotherapy to the use of a person's social environment to effect therapeutic change. Psychotherapy may address spirituality as part of mental life, and some forms are derived from spiritual philosophies, but practices based on treating the spiritual as a separate dimension would not necessarily be considered psychotherapy. Historically psychotherapy has sometimes meant "interpretative" (i.e. Freudian) methods, by contrast with other methods to treat psychiatric disorders such as behaviour modification. Psychotherapy is often dubbed "talking therapy", particularly for a general audience, though not all forms of psychotherapy rely on verbal communication. Children or adults who do not engage in verbal communication (or not in the usual way) are not excluded from psychotherapy; indeed some types are designed for such cases.

## Influence and its tests, classification and assessment

Social influence occurs when one's emotions, opinions, or behaviours are affected by others. Social influence takes many forms and can be seen in conformity, socialization, peer pressure, obedience, leadership, persuasion, sales and marketing. In 1958, Harvard psychologist, Herbert Kelman identified three broad varieties of social influence.

*Compliance is when people appear to agree with others, but actually keep their dissenting opinions private.*

*Identification is when people are influenced by someone who is liked and respected, such as a famous celebrity. Internalization is when people accept a belief or behaviour and agree both publicly and privately.*

Morton Deutsch and Harold Gerard described two psychological needs that lead humans to conform to the expectations of others. These include our need to be right (informational social influence), and our need to be liked (normative social influence). Informational influence (or social proof) is an influence to accept information from another as evidence about reality. Informational influence comes into play when people are uncertain, either because stimuli are intrinsically ambiguous or because there is social disagreement. Normative influence is an influence to conform to the positive expectations of others. In terms of Kelman's typology, normative influence leads to public compliance, whereas informational influence leads to private acceptance.

Compliance is the act of responding favorably to an explicit or implicit request offered by others. Technically, compliance is a change in behaviour but not necessarily attitude- one can comply due to mere obedience, or by otherwise opting to withhold one's private thoughts due to social pressures. According to Kelman's 1958 paper, the satisfaction derived from compliance is due to the social effect of the accepting influence (i.e. people comply for an expected reward or punishment-aversion).

Identification is the changing of attitudes or behaviours due to the influence of someone that is liked. Advertisements that rely upon celebrities to market their products are taking advantage of this phenomenon. The desired relationship that the identifier relates with the behaviour or attitude change is the "reward", according to Kelman.

Internalization is the process of acceptance of a set of norms established by people or groups which are influential to the individual. The individual accepts the influence because the content of the influence accepted is intrinsically rewarding. It is congruent with the individual's value system, and according to Kelman the "reward" of internalization is "the content of the new behaviour".

Conformity is a type of social influence involving a change in behaviour, belief or thinking to align with those of others or to align with normative standards. It is the most common and pervasive form of social influence. Social psychology research in conformity tends to distinguish between two varieties: informational conformity (also called social proof, or "internalization" in Kelman's tems) and normative conformity ("compliance" in Kelman's terms).

In the case of peer pressure, a person is convinced to do something (such as illegal drugs) which they might not want to do, but which they perceive as "necessary" to keep a positive relationship with other people, such as their friends. Conformity from peer pressure generally results from identification within the group members, or from compliance of some members to appease others.

Conformity can be in appearance, or it may be a complete conformity that impacts an individual both publicly and privately.

Compliance (also referred to as acquiescence) demonstrates a public conformity to a group majority or norm while the individual continues to privately disagree or dissent, holding on to their original beliefs or an alternative set of beliefs differing from the majority. Compliance appears as conformity but there is a division between the public and the private self.

Conversion includes the private acceptance that is absent in compliance. The individual's original behaviour, beliefs, or thinking changes to align with that of others (the influencers) both privately as well as publicly. The individual has accepted the behaviour, belief or thinking, and has internalized it, making it their own. Conversion may also refer to individual members of a group who move from their initial (and varied) positions to the same position of others, which may differ from their original positions. The resulting group position may be a hybrid of various aspects of individual initial positions or it may be an alternative independent of the initial positions reached through consensus.

What appears to be conformity may in fact be congruence. Congruence occurs when an individual's behaviour, belief or thinking is already aligned with that of the others and no change occurs.

In situations where conformity (including compliance, conversion and congruence) is absent, there are non-conformity processes such as independence and anti-conformity. Independence (also referred to as dissent) involves an individual, through their actions and/or inactions, or the public expression of their beliefs or thinking, being aligned with their personal standards but inconsistent with that of other members of the group (either all of the group or a majority). Anti-conformity (also referred to as counter-conformity) may appear as independence but lacks alignment with personal standards and is for the purpose of challenging the group. Actions as well as stated opinions and beliefs are often diametrically opposed to that of the group norm or majority. The underlying reasons for this type of behaviour may be rebelliousness/obstinacy or it may be to ensure all alternatives and viewpoints are given due consideration.

Minority influence takes place when a majority is influenced to accept the beliefs or behaviours of a minority. Minority influence can be affected by the sizes of majority and minority groups, the level of consistency of the minority group and situational factors (such as the affluence or social importance of the minority). Minority influence most often operates through informational social influence (as opposed to normative social influence) because the majority may be indifferent to the liking of the minority.

A self-fulfilling prophecy is the prediction that directly or indirectly causes itself to become true, due to a positive feedback between belief and behaviour. A prophecy declared as truth (when it is actually false) may sufficiently influence people, either through fear or logical confusion, so that their reactions ultimately fulfil the once-false prophecy. The term is credited to sociologist Robert K. Merton from his 1948 article.

Reactance is the adoption of a view contrary to the view that they are being pressured to accept, perhaps due to the perceived threat to behavioural freedoms. This behaviour has also been called anticonformity. While the results are the opposite of what the influencer intended, this reactive behaviour is the result of social pressure.[9] It is notable that anticonformity does not necessarily mean independence. In many studies, reactance manifests itself in a deliberate rejection of an influence, even when the influence is clearly correct.

Obedience is a form of social influence that derives from an authority figure. The Milgram Experiment, Zimbardo's Stanford prison experiment, and the Hofling hospital experiment are three particularly well-known experiments on obedience, and they all conclude that humans behave surprisingly obedient in the presence of perceived legitimate authority figures.

Persuasion is the process of guiding oneself or another toward the adoption of some attitude by some rational or symbolic means. Robert Cialdini defined six "weapons of influence": reciprocity, commitment, social proof, authority, liking, and scarcity. These "weapons of influence" attempt to bring about conformity by directed means. Persuasion can occur through appeals to reason or appeals to emotion.

Social Impact Theory was developed by Bibb Latané in 1981. It states that there are three factors which will increase people's likelihood to respond to social influence:

- *Strength: The importance of the influencing group to the individual.*
- *Immediacy: Physical (and temporal) proximity of the influencing group to the individual at the time of the influence attempt. In his work, Robert Cialdini defines six "Weapons of Influence" that can contribute to an individual's propensity to be influenced by a persuader:*
- *Reciprocity: People tend to return a favour.*
- *Commitment and Consistency: People do not like to be self-contradictory. Once they commit to an idea or behaviour, they are averse to changing their minds without good reason.*
- *Social Proof: People will be more open to things they see others doing. For example, seeing others compost their organic waste after finishing a meal may influence them to do so as well.*
- *Authority: People will tend to obey authority figures.*
- *Liking: People are more easily swayed by people they like.*
- *Scarcity: A perceived limitation of resources will generate demand.*

Social Influence is strongest when the group perpetrating it is consistent and committed. Even a single instance of dissent can greatly wane the strength of an influence. For example, in Milgram's first set of obedience experiments, 65% of participants complied with fake authority figures to administer "maximum shocks" to a confederate. In iterations of the Milgram experiment where three people administered shocks (two of whom were confederates), once one confederate disobeyed, only 10% of subjects administered the maximum shocks.

Those perceived as experts may exert social influence as a result of their perceived expertise. This involves credibility, a tool of social influence from which one draws upon the notion of trust. People believe an individual to be credible for a variety of reasons, such as perceived experience, attractiveness, knowledge, etc. Additionally, pressure to maintain one's reputation and not be viewed as fringe may increase the tendency to agree with the group, known as groupthink. Appeals to authority may also especially affect norms of obedience. The compliance of normal humans to authority in the famous Milgram experiment demonstrates the power of perceived authority.

Those with access to the media may use this access in an attempt to influence the public. For example, a politician may use speeches to persuade the public to support issues that he or she does not have the power to impose on the public. This is often referred to as using the "bully pulpit". Likewise, celebrities don't usually possess any political power but are familiar to many of the world's citizens, and therefore possess social status.

Power was found to be one of the most effective reasons as to why an individual feels the need to follow through with what another says to them. If someone of more authority or someone that is believed to be more powerful than the other is an icon or most "popular" within a group, they have the most control over influencing others. For example, in a child's school life, if there are those people who seem to control the perception of the other students at school, then they are most powerful in having a social influence over the other children.

Culture appears to play a role in willingness to conform to a group. Stanley Milgram found that conformity was higher in Norway than in France. This has been attributed to Norway's longstanding tradition of social responsibility, as compared to France's cultural focus on individualism. Japan likewise has a collectivist culture and thus a higher propensity to conform; however, in a 1970 Asch-style study, it was found that, when alienated, Japanese students would be susceptible to anticonformity (giving answers that were incorrect even when the group had coincided on correct answers) one third of the time- significantly higher than has been seen in replications of Asch studies before.

While gender does not significantly affect likelihood to conform, gender roles will in the right conditions. For example, studies from the 1950s and 1960s concluded that women were more likely to conform than men. However, in a 1971 study it was found that there was experimenter bias involved (all of the researchers were male). Studies thereafter found that likelihood to conform was close to equal and that, furthermore, men would conform more often on feminine topics, as women would conform more often on masculine topics- ignorance on a subject can lead to deferral to "social proof".

Emotion and disposition may affect likelihood of conformity or anticonformity. In 2009, a study concluded that fear increases the chance of agreeing with the group, while romance or lust increases the chance of going against the group.

A social network is a social structure made up of nodes (representing individuals or organizations) which are connected (through ties, also called edges, connections, or links) by one or more types of interdependency (such as friendship, common interests or beliefs, sexual relations, or kinship). Social network analysis uses the lens of network theory to view social relationships. Social network analysis as a field has become more prominent since the mid-20th century in determining the channels and effects of social influence. For example, Christakis and Fowler found that social networks transmit states and behaviours such as obesity, smoking, drinking and happiness.

## Short notes of a) Learning and b) Motivation and Influence

a)      Learning theories are conceptual frameworks describing how information is absorbed, processed, and retained during learning. Cognitive, emotional, and environmental influences, as well as prior experience, all play a part in how understanding, or a world view, is acquired or changed and knowledge and skills retained.

Behaviourists look at learning as an aspect of conditioning and will advocate a system of rewards and targets in education. Educators who embrace cognitive theory believe that the definition of learning as a change in behaviour is too narrow and prefer to study the learner rather than their environment and in particular the complexities of human memory. Those who advocate constructivism believe that a learner's ability to learn relies to a large extent on what he already knows and understands, and the acquisition of knowledge should be an individually tailored process of construction. Transformative learning theory focuses upon the often-necessary change that is required in a learner's preconceptions and world view.

Outside the realm of educational psychology, techniques to directly observe the functioning of the brain during the learning process, such as event-related potential and functional magnetic resonance imaging, are used in educational neuroscience. As of 2012, such studies are beginning to support a theory of multiple intelligences, where learning is seen as the interaction between dozens of different functional areas in the brain each with their own individual strengths and weaknesses in any particular human learner.

b)      Most motivation theorists assume that motivation is involved in the performance of all learned responses; that is, a learned behaviour will not occur unless it is energized.  The major question among psychologists, in general, is whether motivation is a primary or secondary influence on behaviour. That is, are changes in behaviour better explained by principles of environmental/ecological influences, perception, memory, cognitive development, emotion, explanatory style, or personality or are concepts unique to motivation more pertinent.
For example, it is known that people respond to increasingly complex or novel events (or stimuli) in the environment up to a point and then the rate of responding decreases.  This inverted-U-shaped curve of behaviour is well-known and widely acknowledged (e.g., Yerkes & Dodson, 1908).  However, the major issue is one of explaining this phenomenon.  This is a conditioning (is the individual behaving because

of past classical or operant conditioning), another type of external motivation such as social or ecological, an internal motivational process (e.g., cognition, emotion, or self-regulation).

In general, explanations regarding the source(s) of motivation can be categorized as either extrinsic (outside the person) or intrinsic (internal to the person).  Intrinsic sources and corresponding theories can be further subcategorized as either body/physical, mind/mental (i.e., cognitive/thinking, affective/emotional, conative/volitional) or transpersonal/spiritual.

## Gestalt Therapy and its implementation in the therapeutic process

Gestalt therapy is an existential/experiential form of psychotherapy that emphasizes personal responsibility, and that focuses upon the individual's experience in the present moment, the therapist–client relationship, the environmental and social contexts of a person's life, and the self-regulating adjustments people make as a result of their overall situation.
Gestalt therapy was developed by Fritz Perls, Laura Perls and Paul Goodman in the 1940s and 1950s. Edwin Nevis described Gestalt therapy as "a conceptual and methodological base from which helping professionals can craft their practice". In the same volume, Joel Latner stated that Gestalt therapy is built upon two central ideas: that the most helpful focus of psychotherapy is the experiential present moment, and that everyone is caught in webs of relationships; thus, it is only possible to know ourselves against the background of our relationships to others. The historical development of Gestalt therapy (described below) discloses the influences that generated these two ideas. Expanded, they support the four chief theoretical constructs (explained in the theory and practice section) that comprise Gestalt theory, and that guide the practice and application of Gestalt therapy.

Gestalt therapy was forged from various influences upon the lives of its founders during the times in which they lived, including: the new physics, Eastern religion, existential phenomenology, Gestalt psychology, psychoanalysis, experimental theatre, as well as systems theory and field theory. Gestalt therapy rose from its beginnings in the middle of the 20th century to rapid and widespread popularity during the decade of the 1960s and early 1970s. During the '70s and '80s Gestalt therapy training centers spread globally; but they were, for the most part, not aligned with formal academic settings. As the cognitive revolution eclipsed Gestalt theory in psychology, many came to believe Gestalt was an anachronism. Because Gestalt therapists disdained the positivism underlying what they perceived to be the concern of research, they largely ignored the need to utilize research to further develop Gestalt theory and Gestalt therapy practice (with a few exceptions like Les Greenberg, see the interview: "Validating Gestalt" However, the new century has seen a sea of change in attitudes toward research and Gestalt practice.

Gestalt therapy is not identical with Gestalt psychology but Gestalt psychology influenced the development of Gestalt therapy to a large extent.

Gestalt therapy focuses on process (what is actually happening) over content (what is being talked about). The emphasis is on what is being done, thought, and felt at the present moment (the phenomenality of both client and therapist), rather than on what was, might be, could be, or should have been. Gestalt therapy is a method of awareness practice (also called "mindfulness" in other clinical domains), by which perceiving, feeling, and acting are understood to be conducive to interpreting, explaining, and conceptualizing (the hermeneutics of experience). This distinction between direct experiences versus indirect or secondary interpretation is developed in the process of therapy. The client learns to become aware of what he or she is doing and that triggers the ability to risk a shift or change.

The objective of Gestalt therapy is to enable the client to become more fully and creatively alive and to become free from the blocks and unfinished business that may diminish satisfaction, fulfilment, and growth, and to experiment with new ways of being. For this reason Gestalt therapy falls within the category of humanistic psychotherapies. Because Gestalt therapy includes perception and the meaning-making processes by which experience forms, it can also be considered a cognitive approach. Because Gestalt therapy relies on the contact between therapist and client, and because a relationship can be considered to be contact over time, Gestalt therapy can be considered a relational or interpersonal approach. Because Gestalt therapy appreciates the larger picture which is the complex situation involving multiple influences in a complex situation, it can be considered a multi-systemic approach. Because the processes of Gestalt therapy are experimental, involving action, Gestalt therapy can be considered both a paradoxical and an experiential/experimental approach.

When Gestalt therapy is compared to other clinical domains, a person can find many matches, or points of similarity. "Probably the clearest case of consilience is between gestalt therapy's field perspective and the various organismic and field theories that proliferated in neuroscience, medicine, and physics in the early and mid-20th century. Within social science there is a consilience between gestalt field theory and systems or ecological psychotherapy; between the concept of dialogical relationship and object relations, attachment theory, client-centered therapy and the transference-oriented approaches; between the existential, phenomenological, and hermeneutical aspects of gestalt therapy and the constructivist aspects of cognitive therapy; and between gestalt therapy's commitment to awareness and the natural processes of healing and mindfulness, acceptance and Buddhist techniques adopted by cognitive behavioural therapy."

## Cognitive Behaviour Therapy and its clinical importance

Cognitive–behavioural therapy (CBT) is a short term, problem-focused psychosocial intervention. Evidence from randomised controlled trials and meta analyses shows that it is an effective intervention for depression, panic disorder, generalised anxiety and obsessive–compulsive disorder (Department of Health, 2001). Increasing evidence indicates its usefulness in a growing range of other psychiatric disorders such as health anxiety/hypochondriasis, social phobia, schizophrenia and bipolar disorders. CBT is also of proven benefit to patients who attend psychiatric clinics (Paykel et al, 1999). The model is fully compatible with the use of medication, and studies examining depression have tended to confirm that CBT used together with antidepressant medication is more effective than either treatment alone (Blackburn et al, 1981) and that CBT treatment may lead to a reduction in future relapse (Evans et al, 1992). Generic CBT skills provide a readily accessible model for patient assessment and management and can usefully inform general

clinical skills in everyday practice. CBT can be offered as an integrated part of a biopsychosocial assessment and management approach, but there are certain situations in which it should be particularly considered;

-The patient prefers to use psychological interventions, either alone or in addition to medication

-The target problems for CBT (extreme, unhelpful thinking; reduced activity; avoidant
or unhelpful behaviours) are present

-No improvement or only partial improvement has occurred on medication
-Side-effects prevent a sufficient dose of medication from being taken over an adequate period

-Significant psychosocial problems (e.g. relationship problems, difficulties at work or unhelpful behaviours such as self-cutting or alcohol misuse) are present that will not be adequately addressed by medication alone. Effective psychosocial interventions share certain characteristics. They provide: a focus on current problems of relevance to the patient; a clear underlying model, structure or plan to the treatment being offered; and delivery that is built on an effective relationship with the practitioner. CBT is founded on these principles and is essentially a psychoeducational form of psychotherapy. Its purpose is for patients to learn new skills of self-management that they will then put into practice in everyday life. It adopts a collaborative stance that encourages patients to work on changing how they feel by putting into practice what they have learned.

## 3. *Chiropractic*

### Contraindications for Chiropractic Practice

*Ruptured disc:* When evaluating for a disc injury, the chiropractor will want to rule out an extruded (or ruptured) disc and will refer patient out for an MRI if he or she suspects that the disc is torn. Ruptured discs CAN be successfully treated by chiropractors, but the methods of treatment will be unique to this condition.

*Cardiovascular problems:* When considering the potential for cardiovascular issues, the chiropractor will look for predisposing factors based upon patient's family history. The chiropractor will also ask about whether patient is a smoker, are on steroids or blood thinning medications, and (if female patient) whether patient is on birth control medications. It is important to perform special tests to evaluate the vertebral arteries (the small arteries in the neck which run alongside and within a portion of the vertebrae).

*Bone weakness:* The chiropractor will check for the structural integrity of the bones prior to SMT. If patient has Osteoporosis, Rheumatoid or Osteoarthritic Degenerative Disease, special methods of SMT can be performed safely. An instrument adjusting technique (Pro-Adjuster, Sigma Instruments, Pulstar Instruments) can be safely used.

*Abnormalities:* It is important to check the spine for congenital abnormalities or space-occupying problems which could (very rarely) include tumors or disease.

*Infection:* Checking vital signs is important, especially temperature, to rule out the possibility of an infection.

*Problems with visceral organs:* Symptoms from the viscera and internal organs can mimic musculoskeletal symptoms, and may require immediate medical or emergency room referral. (Gall bladder pain or an aortic aneurysm are examples of mimicked spinal pain.)

*Muscle spasms:* If there is an acute spasm of a muscle, SMT in that immediate area will not be appropriate.

*Certain pain patterns:* We won't perform SMT into a spinal region if patient shows symptoms into BOTH arms or BOTH legs without an MRI first. This is important if other orthopaedic and neurological tests are positive.

*Congenital scoliosis:* SMT is not going to decrease the progressive effects of congenital juvenile idiopathic scoliosis.

*Surgical hardware:* It is not allowed to perform SMT into surgical fusion hardware, especially if the surgery was recent.

## The beliefs in subluxations between straight and mixers

The group of chiropractors who believe in subluxations can be subdivided into two groups, the "straights" and the"mixers." The straights follow Palmer's doctrine that subluxations of the vertebrae can cause or contribute to most disorders, but they do not claim to be able to diagnose or treat diseases -only to detect and cure subluxations. Only about 15 percent of all chiropractors can be called "straight" chiropractors.

Straight chiropractor's consider their scope of practice limited to:

- *The anatomy of the spine and immediate articulations*
- *The condition of vertebral subluxation*
- *Addressing vertebral subluxations*
- *Educating patients and advising them about subluxations.*
- *Mixers believe that diseases can develop from other causes, like bacteria and viruses. But they believe that subluxations affect the body's health by lowering resistance to disease. The deviation or malposition of a spinal vertebra may cause a neurological imbalance within the body, setting the stage for a lowered resistance.*

Mixers comprise the majority of practitioners. Their practice extends beyond the narrow focus on vertebral subluxation. They use a wider range of modalities as well as concepts from diverse health care traditions in their practice. Many integrate methods from other traditions. The most common are: nutritional supplementation, vitamins, homeopathic drugs, and nutritional advice. Some integrate Chinese medicine, Ayurveda, naturopathy, homeopathy, massage or bodywork, mind/body approaches, or other healing methods into their offerings. Individual chiropractors often develop their own unique reputation and synthesis of different traditions.

## The role of John Mc Timoney in founding the Mc Timoney method of chiropractic

John MC Timoney was born in 1914 in Birmingham, UK. Whilst working as a farm labourer during World War Two, John McTimoney fell from a ladder. After this fall walking became difficult as did using both arms. X-Rays did not reveal the cause of the problem. Fortunately, he was introduced to Chiropractic Doctor Ashford in Birmingham who had been trained by the founder of Chiropractic, DD Palmer, in the USA. John McTimoney's first Chiropractic treatment consisted of a single adjustment to the top vertebrae in his neck, C1, also known as the "Atlas". This is the so-called "hole-in-one" adjustment, after which John McTimoney was able to walk five miles home. Previously, this would have been impossible. He continued to receive treatment for three years and he longed to become a Chiropractor but there was at that time no Chiropractic college in the UK.

Eventually, in 1948, John McTimoney was able to become the second pupil of Chiropractic Doctor Mary Walker and he qualified in 1950. Mary Walker, 1880-1958, had started her professional career as a nursing matron and she had converted her north Oxfordshire house into a nursing home. After a car accident she was treated for spinal injury by a Palmer-trained Chiropractor. She was very impressed and in the 1930s she went to the U.S. to train with BJ Palmer, the son of the founder of Chiropractic, DD Palmer. Mary Walker was a star pupil. She returned to the UK in 1936 to set up her own practice in Oxford. In addition to Chiropractic technique she also used Bach flower remedies, homeopathy, and radionics. Also, at first as a diagnostic aid, she used a neurocalometer, a device to detect inflammation. However, she came to the opinion that such devices were less effective than thought and that palpation was a quicker and more accurate way of detecting skeletal misalignment. Her first pupil, starting in 1947, was Joan Nind. Her second and last pupil was John McTimoney. He couldn't even pay his fees, but Mary Walker trained him anyway. Mary Walker had hoped to establish a Chiropractic college but this dream was only to be realised by her student, John McTimoney.

John McTimoney qualified in 1950 and started his own practice in 1951 in Banbury. Mary Walker helped him to set up, providing him with essential equipment he could not of otherwise afford. For a while he had to supplement his income teaching carpentry at a local school. One of his first patients was his wife, Hilda. She had a serious problem with her arm and John McTimoney was able to treat her and enable her to continue her work as a silver-smith. John McTimoney's reputation grew and he began to attract patients from all over the UK and abroad.

In 1954, John McTimoney formulated a method of Chiropractic analysis and treatment for animals. He was the first UK Chiropractor to do this. Treating animals started when a horse owning patient had to cancel an appointment because an eleven year old horse was lame. The owner suggested John McTimoney have a look at the animal which, after Chiropractic treatment, went on to have a good recovery. From this beginning, John McTimoney developed a whole-body treatment for horses, dogs, cats and cows. Unfortunately, this new approach to treatment aggrieved the veterinary profession on the basis that UK law forbade non-veterinary surgeons from treating animals. A court case started to develop as John McTimoney defended his position, claiming he was not practising as a veterinary surgeon but had evolved an entirely new Chiropractic treatment. Quentin Hogg (later Lord Hailsham) was tasked to act for John McTimoney. The cost was to be borne by prominent horsemen David Broome and Ted Edgar. However, the stress of the case and John McTimoney's overworking led to John McTimoney having a heart attack in the very week the case was meant to be heard. McTimoney Therapy is a gentle yet highly effective full body treatment for spinal and skeletal misalignment. Practiced for over 30 years, this distinctive technique offers an alternative to many forms of chiropractic and osteopathy.

In McTimoney Therapy 'cracking' and 'popping' sounds are rare. This is because the adjustments are highly specific, using the speed and dexterity of their delivery to correct misalignment, rather than a more vigorous approach. Consequently, the majority of patients find the treatment comfortable and pain free to receive.

The entire skeleton is routinely assessed for misalignment to determine the true source of any pain symptoms. The pain experienced and the source of pain are not necessarily one and the same. This can occur as a result of compensations automatically made by the body when alignment is lost. For example, it is not uncommon for symptoms in the back and the neck to originate in an unbalanced pelvis. McTimoney Therapy aims to treat the cause of the problem, not just the symptom. As McTimoney Therapy delivers a full body treatment, it can achieve excellent results for any of the body's joints; from those of the skull right down to the fingers and toes.

The spine and pelvis (the foundation of the spine) are given particular attention, as correct alignment of the spine is crucial to the optimum function of your nervous system. Every delicate fibre transmitting, every sensation from the body to the brain and every instruction from the brain to the body's muscles and organs travel via the spine.

Many conditions are often helped by McTimoney Therapy. These include;

- *-Back, neck and shoulder pain*
- *-Pain, discomfort and stiffness in joints and bones*
- *-Headaches / Migraines*
- *-Muscular aches and pains*
- *-Sciatica and disc complications*
- *-Numbness and tingling*
- *-Whiplash injury*
- *-Sports injuries*
- *-Repetitive strain injury*

## The advantages of Chiropractic over the diseases like Infantile Colic and Chronic Migraines

Infantile colic can be as troublesome for the parent as the child experiencing the condition. Characterized by a multitude of symptoms, the child suffering from infantile colic does not usually respond to simple comforting methods and exhibits periodic fussiness that can last over hours or days. In many cases the infant appears to be in pain and will pull up his/her legs. At times the child's abdomen will be hard and distended. Occasionally the passage of flatus will give relief, yet these attacks may last for hours. To make matters more complicated, this condition rarely responds to traditional health care. This leaves many parents troubled as an infant's episodes of crying and fussiness persist. Two chiropractic studies relating to infantile colic are of particular interest. The first study was done by a group of Danish chiropractors who revealed positive results when spinal adjustments were given to a group of infants with colic symptoms. A second study involving a group of 316 infants diagnosed with colic reported 94% successful resolution within the first two weeks of chiropractic care.

Although chiropractic care does not treat the symptoms of colic specifically, Chiropractors have found after adjusting hundreds of babies that most will respond within the first few weeks. Nerve supply is vital to the proper function of every system of the body, including the stomach, intestines, and other abdominal organs. Any vertebral subluxation causing interference to the nerves in this area could adversely affect gastric function and result in discomfort, gas and other colic symptoms. As the infant with colic responds to chiropractic care, parents usually note that the child sleeps for longer periods without fussing, and requires less comforting.

As chiropractic helps to restore normal function in child's nervous system, infant's digestive tract and other related organs have a better opportunity to receive nerve supply from the brain, bringing it back to full normal potential.

Chronic Migraine There aren't many large studies on the value of chiropractic treatment in managing migraines. One study examined chiropractic treatment for different types of headaches, including migraines. The study combined the results of 22 studies, which had more than 2,600 patients total. The studies show that chiropractic treatment may serve as a good preventive treatment for migraines. Another trial found that 22 percent of people who had chiropractic treatment saw the number of attacks drop 90 percent. In that same study, 49 percent said they had a significant reduction in pain intensity. One study of 127 migraine sufferers in Australia found that those that received chiropractic treatment had fewer attacks and needed to take less medication. The 1999 study found that more than 80 percent of the patients blamed stress for leading to their migraine attacks. Therefore researchers believe chiropractic care might physically help reduce the body's reaction to stress.

## Chiropractic increasing energy

The body's energy flow will become blocked if the spinal bones are locked AND when the neck and back muscles are tense. Sore, tense muscles are the result of joints not moving freely, causing all the muscles around the joint to contract and spasm. The water flow through the hose is interrupted and blocked. It's the same thing with the nerve supply running through the back. By repositioning the joints to their proper place, the muscles relax and energy can flow freely through the body. A lot of chiropractic patients report feeling an increase in energy, as well as an overall sense of relaxation after receiving an adjustment.

## Treatment in cases of Asthma and Back Pain

 According to the American Academy of Allergy, Asthma, and Immunology, "one in 12 people (about 25 million or 8% of the U.S. population) had asthma in 2009." With such a high prevalence, asthma is undoubtedly a disease that needs to be looked at. While traditional solutions like inhalers and prescription medications are commonplace in the treatment of asthma, chiropractic care should also be considered as viable options. Asthma can occur as a result of environmental factors including air pollutants (dust, smoke), or because of emotional stress or related illness. It leads to shortness of breath, wheezing, irritating cough, and can even progress into a full blown attack in which an individual requires an emergency inhaler or even medical attention. These things occur because asthma causes the lungs and airway to constrict, and inflammation makes it difficult for the body to effectively conduct and deliver oxygen to needy cells.

Many individuals with asthma have resolved to maintenance of the illness, using inhalers and medication. But chiropractic care has been shown to help improve the condition with regular treatment, and provides an alternative to these traditional therapies. Chiropractic treatment involves the realignment of the spine and therefore the nerves, which play a role in every function the body carries out. Accordingly, chiropractic manipulation can adjust an individual and eliminate obstruction during nerve impulse conduction to the lungs and airway. By restoring the body to its natural state of alignment, nerves can function as they should, allowing organs (namely lungs) to function as they should. In addition to bettering nerve function, chiropractic care can also benefit asthma sufferers by fixing musculoskeletal alignment problems in the ribcage and spine. In doing so, the thoracic cavity is free to expand as it should, and take in the air the body requires to live. Because asthma is such a widespread disease, it is important to look at all the treatment options, as some individuals respond better to certain methods. Chiropractic care for the treatment of asthma is a non-invasive option for patients who have either tried other unsuccessful routes, or patients who are looking for alternatives to medications. In addition to helping patients achieve optimum alignment, chiropractors may also consult them on ways to reduce exposure to asthma-inducing allergens or triggers. Lifestyle changes like these can also be an asset in the asthma treatment process.

Many studies have concluded that manual therapies commonly used by chiropractors are generally effective for the treatment of back pain, as well as for treatment of lumbar herniated disc for radiculopathy and neck pain, among other conditions.

In fact, when patients with non-specific chronic low back pain are treated by chiropractors, the long-term outcome is enhanced by obtaining maintenance spinal manipulation after the initial intensive manipulative therapy.

## Philosophy of Chiropractic on holistic concept

Chiropractic has a philosophy on healing and health which differs from the traditional medical view. Chiropractors approach health in a holistic manner. In other words, chiropractors evaluate the entire person as a whole when assessing and treating a patient's health ailment or disease, rather than focusing solely on a symptom or specific area of the body. They know that the body is able to maintain and heal itself in most cases. We also know that true health is not achieved through the ingestion of chemicals or the cutting away of diseased tissues. Instead, health is something that comes from within and is inherent to our body. The chiropractic treatment is based upon the understanding that circumstances occur which may require medical intervention, but ultimately, it is the body that conducts and manages the process of healing and not the doctor or externally applied forces. When the chiropractor corrects spinal abnormalities and eliminates spinal and nerve irritation and interference, pain is alleviated and the body's inborn healing capabilities are set into motion.

## Advantages of chiropractic over premenstrual syndrome

Premenstrual syndrome (PMS) is a collection of symptoms linked to the menstrual cycle and usually occur 1 to 2 weeks prior to your period. The symptoms usually stop after you start menstruating. For some women, PMS is just a monthly nag. For other women, however, it can be so agonizing it makes it incredibly difficult to even make it throughout the day. PMS goes away when your monthly periods stop, such as pregnancy or menopause. Up to 90 percent of menstruating women report having one or more premenstrual symptoms, and 10 to 20 percent report disabling, debilitating symptoms. While chiropractic care isn't a treatment for PMS, many women experiencing spinal distortions have seen an improvement in their reproductive health while under chiropractic care. Restoring normality and restoring a functioning nervous system helps the entire body work the way it is supposed to.

PMS was originally seen as something women made up. Women who reported its symptoms were often being told it was "all in their head". If there's evidence of nerve compromise to the reproductive organs, chiropractic care helps. Chiropractic care is shown to be helpful in relieving many PMS symptoms in several studies when receiving two to three adjustments during the weeks leading up to the onset of the menstrual cycle.

## Chiropractic in paediatric practice

Chiropractic care for children offers the family a solid foundation for wellness. Throughout pregnancy, birth, and childhood, the chiropractic lifestyle offers choices and benefits for a greater health and well-being. The ICPA has initiated a ground breaking study on the safety and effectiveness of chiropractic care for children. The preliminary results are outstanding and show that chiropractic care is safe for children. Even more significant is that parents reported three unexpected improvements with their child's care: Improved sleeping, improved behaviour and attitude, improved immune system function. In general, chiropractic care for children is painless, except in cases where the child has an actual injury. In these areas, the child may be sensitive to touch; however, once the adjustment has been made and the area can heal more effectively, the sensitivity is alleviated. Overall, most parents report that their children enjoy their spinal adjustments.

## Key principles of Chiropractic: a) The Vitalistic Principle and b) the cause of illness

Vitalism is a philosophy (way of thinking about life) which understands that someone or some intelligent energy source or some non-material force or inborn power makes us alive and coordinates all functions of life.

The truth about how the body works is simple: We are self-healing self-regulating organisms. Health and adaptation comes from inside us. This inborn innate intelligence sustains every vital aspect of life in your body: including growth, healing, cellular function, reproduction, immune system, breathing, balance, heartbeat, etc. Vitalism is foundational to everything we do at Chiropractic. Chiropractic restores vital connection to that innate power source so you patients fully express life to the potential.

Chiropractic tradition holds that much of illness occurs as a result of disturbances in the nervous system. Such disturbances are caused by derangements of the musculoskeletal structure. These disturbances may cause or aggravate disease in various parts or functions of the body. Subluxations occur as a normal part of living in any culture. Our bodies were not designed to sit for long periods of time. The modern sedentary lifestyle consisting of little exercise and long periods of sitting, either at desks, in cars, or at home, puts an unnatural strain on the spine and contributes to subluxations. The spine does not receive the degree of daily movement with which it evolved. Modern lifestyles often impede a normal, healthful degree of flexibility. Many chiropractors also hold that health is further compromised by other aspects of lifestyle, such as inadequate nutrition, pollution and chronic stress. All these factors together create a situation in which the flow of vital force through the nervous system is impaired at a time when it is needed to be at its optimum. This results in the variety of chronic and degenerative illnesses we face today. Chiropractic and many other natural health disciplines recognize that to be truly healthy and alive you must be a clear conduit to your inner wisdom (also referred to as your "source," the "wisdom of the body", your "inner doctor", your innate (inborn) intelligence and other terms).

The goal of chiropractic is to help patients better connect to their sources so they self-healing-system may work its miracles. A complete disconnection from the source results in death; a partial disconnection results in disease or disharmony. Many people are in this state; with less than 100% connection they are less than fully alive.

## 4. *Medicinal Herbalism*

### Two important Endocrinal Disorders in brief

The endocrine system is a network of glands that produce and release hormones that help control many important body functions, including the body's ability to change calories into energy that powers cells and organs. The endocrine system influences heartbeat, bones and tissues grow and sexuality. It plays a vital role in whether or not you develop diabetes, thyroid disease, growth disorders, sexual dysfunction, and a host of other hormone-related disorders. Each gland of the endocrine system releases specific hormones into your bloodstream. These hormones travel through your blood to other cells and help control or coordinate many body processes. There are different gland types as follows:

*Adrenal glands:* Two glands that sit on top of the kidneys that release the hormone cortisol.
*Hypothalamus:* A part of the lower middle brain that tells the pituitary gland when to release hormones.
*Ovaries:* The female reproductive organs that release eggs and produce sex hormones.
*Islet cells in the pancreas:* Cells in the pancreas control the release of the hormones insulin and glucagon.
*Parathyroid:* Four tiny glands in the neck that play a role in bone development.
*Pineal gland:* A gland found near the mediastinum of the brain that may be linked to sleep patterns.
*Pituitary gland:* A gland found at the base of brain behind the sinuses. It is often called the "master gland" because it influences many other glands, especially the thyroid. Problems with the pituitary gland can affect bone growth, a woman's menstrual cycles, and the release of breast milk.
*Testes:* The male reproductive glands that produce sperm and sex hormones.
*Thymus:* A gland in the upper chest that helps to develop the body's immune system early in life.

*Thyroid:* A butterfly-shaped gland in the front of the neck that controls metabolism.

Even the slightest hiccup with the function of one or more of these glands can throw off the delicate balance of hormones in your body and lead to an endocrine disorder, or endocrine disease.

Endocrine disorders are typically grouped into two categories: Endocrine disease that results when a gland produces too much or too little of an endocrine hormone, called a hormone imbalance. Endocrine disease due to the development of lesions (such as nodules or tumors) in the endocrine system, which may or may not affect hormone levels. The endocrine's feedback system helps control the balance of hormones in the bloodstream. If your body has too much or too little of a certain hormone, the feedback system signals the proper gland or glands to correct the problem. A hormone imbalance may occur if this feedback system has trouble keeping the right level of hormones in the bloodstream, or if your body doesn't clear them out of the bloodstream properly. Increased or decreased levels of endocrine hormone may be caused by:

- *A problem with the endocrine feedback system*
- *Disease*
- *Failure of a gland to stimulate another gland to release hormones (for example, a problem with the hypothalamus can disrupt hormone production in the pituitary gland)*
- *A genetic disorder, such as multiple endocrine neoplasia (MEN) or congenital hypothyroidism*
- *Infection*
- *Injury to an endocrine gland*
- *Tumor of an endocrine gland*

Most endocrine tumors and nodules (lumps) are noncancerous. They usually do not spread to other parts of the body. However, a tumor or nodule on the gland may interfere with the gland's hormone production. There are many different types of endocrine disorders. Diabetes is the most common endocrine disorder diagnosed in the U.S.

*Adrenal insufficiency:* The adrenal gland releases too little of the hormone cortisol and sometimes, aldosterone. Symptoms include fatigue, stomach upset, dehydration, and skin changes. Addison's disease is a type of adrenal insufficiency.

*Cushing's disease*: Overproduction of a pituitary gland hormone leads to an overactive adrenal gland. A similar condition called Cushing's syndrome may occur in people, particularly children, who take high doses of corticosteroid medications.

*Gigantism (acromegaly) and other growth hormone problems:* If the pituitary gland produces too much growth hormone, a child's bones and body parts may grow abnormally fast. If growth hormone levels are too low, a child can stop growing in height.

*Hyperthyroidism:* The thyroid gland produces too much thyroid hormone, leading to weight loss, fast heart rate, sweating, and nervousness. The most common cause for an overactive thyroid is an autoimmune disorder called Grave's disease.

## Medicated Massage and Hydrotherapy

Hydrotherapy is an important, time-tested adjunct to hands-on modalities. This use of water to heat, cool, stimulate, relax, and detoxify the human body has been used for thousands of years and by many cultures throughout the world. Native-American sweat lodges, Indian ayurvedic steam treatments, Greek and Roman hot and cold baths, Finnish saunas, and Japanese hot springs are just a few examples.

Few massage therapists are aware that many hydrotherapy treatments can be performed in the office or work space without investing in large and expensive equipment. Simple treatments that involve ice massage, hot packs, friction treatments, contrast applications, and compresses are inexpensive, effective, require little time, and are often preferred by patients. Many hydrotherapy treatments can make a massage therapists work easier. For example, ice applications reduce inflammation and help treat trigger points; heating treatments enhance the flexibility of scar tissue; friction treatments stimulate the skin, increase localized blood flow and may reduce muscle tension; warm baths relieve stress and warm the entire body before a session; and paraffin dips warm and soothe arthritic joints. Hydrotherapy self-care can also be introduced by massage therapists as a "take home" after the session to encourage patient follow-up, thus enhance the effects of the bodywork. Massage and hydrotherapy can relieve discomfort and pain, stimulate the flow of blood and lymph, and make connective tissue easier to stretch. If patients are too hot or too cold, hydrotherapy treatments can make them more comfortable before or during a massage session. Hydrotherapy treatments can also stimulate the skin in different ways—from the body-hugging sensation of being surrounded by water, the thermal sensations of warm or cool, or the scratchy feeling of friction treatment.

Assisting neuromuscular tension and toning up the nervous system, medicated massage helps to revitalize the vital force and enhance the immunity mechanisms, removes the accumulated body wastes, poisons, foreign substances and it helps the body in cleansing and regenerating by stimulation of glands and organs, it aids to regulate the blood vessels, lymphatics, muscles, tissues, tendons, bones, ligaments from all undue pressure, possible deformities and obstructions,  to develop weak muscles, tendons, ligaments and other necessary adjustments, it improves coordination of movement, increases mobility of joints and defective postures. In sum we have to know, that physical medicine corrects all discoverable abnormalities of the body in all forms. Physiotherapy with its broad field of inducement and a long history back to first Egyptian manuscripts explaining scientific massage is one of the most popular naturopathic methods, often recommended through primary care physicians and as part of postoperative clinical treatments.

## The determinants of Positive Health

Positive health describes a state beyond the mere absence of disease and is definable and measurable. Positive health can be operationalised by a combination of excellent status on biological, subjective, and functional measures. By mining existing longitudinal studies, we can test the hypothesis that positive health predicts increased longevity (correcting for quality of life), decreased health costs, better mental health in aging, and better prognosis when illness strikes. Those aspects of positive health which specifically predict these outcomes then become targets for new interventions and refinements of protocol. It proposes that the field of positive health has direct parallels to the field of positive psychology, parallels that suggest that a focus on health rather than illness will be cost saving and lifesaving. Finally, it suggests a different mode of science, the Copenhagen-Medici model, used to found positive psychology, as an appropriate way of beginning the flagship explorations for positive health.

In conclusion, it is suggested that the exploration of positive mental health, as opposed to mere absence of mental illness, has proved fruitful in positive psychology. Positive health, as opposed to mere absence of positive physical illness, has long been ignored scientifically. Positive health is not only a desirable in its own right, however; it is also a likely buffer against physical and mental illness. It is believed that positive health can be defined and operationalised. Once operationalised, positive health is a potential predictor of longevity, health costs, mental health in aging, and prognosis when illness strikes. These flagship predictive studies will, if successful, find specific subjective, functional, and biological variables that mediate longevity, mental health, and lower health costs in general, and better prognosis in specific disorders. It is believed that the definitional and predictive studies will provide the necessary groundwork for an expansive exploration of positive health. The most expansive and important implication of these flagship studies will be the interventions and refinements of protocol that follow; novel and inexpensive interventions that build the specific elements of positive health become candidates for the treatment and prevention of both positive physical and mental illness.

## Medicinal Herbalism and its modus operandi

Herbalism (also herbology or herbal medicine) is the use of plants for medicinal purposes, and the study of botany for such use. Plants have been the basis for medical treatments through much of human history, and such traditional medicine is still widely practiced today. Modern medicine recognizes herbalism as a form of alternative medicine, as the practice of herbalism is not strictly based on evidence gathered using the scientific method. Modern medicine, does, however, make use of many plant-derived compounds as the basis for evidence-tested pharmaceutical drugs, phytotherapy, and phytochemistry works to apply modern standards of effectiveness testing to herbs and medicines that are derived from natural sources. The scope of herbal medicine is sometimes extended to include fungal and bee products, as well as minerals, shells and certain animal parts.

The World Health Organization (WHO) estimates that 80 percent of the population of some Asian and African countries presently use herbal medicine for some aspect of primary health care. Pharmaceuticals are prohibitively expensive for most of the world's population, half of whom lived on less than $2 U.S. per day in 2002. In comparison, herbal medicines can be grown from seed or gathered from nature for little or no cost.

Many of the pharmaceuticals currently available to physicians have a long history of use as herbal remedies, including opium, aspirin, digitalis, and quinine. According to the World Health Organization, approximately 25% of modern drugs used in the United States have been derived from plants. At least 7,000 medical compounds in the modern pharmacopoeia are derived from plants. Among the 120 active compounds currently isolated from the higher plants and widely used in modern medicine today, 80% show a positive correlation between their modern therapeutic use and the traditional use of the plants from which they are derived.

## The methods of covering, drying and storing herbs

It is important to prepare Herbs for storage as soon as possible. Every herbalist has his or her own techniques and favourite methods of storing herbs, and some of them are quite simple. The most popular means of preserving herbs is by drying. In removing the moisture from the cellular structure of the plant, you trap the "active principles," or therapeutically useful chemicals, inside. Also, the plant is impervious to mold, disease, and other problems. Dried herbs can—depending on the species—be stored for up to five years with no loss of potency. Basically, there are two methods of drying, both of which have certain advantages and disadvantages. The quicker—and more common—method is indoor oven drying. The other method, which some herbalists find preferable, is outdoor frame-drying. Oven Drying: The main advantage of oven drying is the way in which it saves time. Herbs that would normally take up to six weeks to dry naturally can be dried within an hour indoors.

The herbs should be placed neatly, side by side, on a clean, dry oven tray. A piece of aluminium foil should be placed over the tray, with the reflective side facing in. The foil should then be nipped to the edges of the tray, leaving a small gap to allow moisture to escape.

Place the tray into the oven, which should be set on the lowest temperature (150°F). Remove the tray every 15 minutes and turn the herbs over to ensure that the moisture is drawn out evenly from all sides of the plant. If moisture is drawn out through one side more rapidly than the other, burning may occur. Do not allow plants to burn to a dark brown or black colour. When this happens, the potency is destroyed completely and the plant is useless.

There are two disadvantages to oven drying. First, it is extremely easy to over-dry or burn the herbage. Remember, you are trying to dry the herb, not cook it. When the leaves or peals crumble gently in your hand without powdering, and some or all of original colour is intact, then the plant is dried sufficiently. The second disadvantage of oven-drying is that, for various reasons, the herbs lose between 1/3 to 1/2 of their original potency, compared to their outdoor-dried equivalents which only lose around 1/4.

Frame Drying: Although this method is more time-consuming than oven drying, it is often preferred by experienced herbalists, as the loss of potency is somewhat less.

For frame-drying, you will need a small wooden or metal box about 3' square, with a glass lie. The base of the frame should be lined with aluminium foil, leaving a small, sheltered hole for ventilation. Herbs selected for drying should be placed on the aluminium foil, and the lid closed afterwards. The plants should be turned once a day until dry.

The frame should, of course, be situated in an area that receives a reasonable amount of sunlight. It should be absolutely watertight, and all herbs placed in it should be dried gently with a cloth first. One damp herb placed in the frame may be sufficient to turn the entire batch moldy. Frame drying may take anything between three to six weeks.

Having successfully dried the selected herbs, it is an effort to decide the method of storing them. This is largely determined by the eventual form in which the herb is to be administered. Ointments, for instance, are normally made from finely powdered herbs, while tinctures are usually made by submerging the whole root or leaves in alcohol. As a rough guide, it should be suggested that the leaves, bark, and stem are best comminuted (ground), while root, petals, and seeds are best stored whole. Be sure that your herbs are thoroughly dried before storage.

## A holistic prescription for Migraine and IBS

IBS with its symptoms may be so severe that patients can't leave the house and we call it a "functional," or "psychosomatic," disease — meaning that it's all in the head.

It's a very real problem for the 60 million people — that's 20 percent of Americans — who have irritable bowel syndrome (IBS). These people are plagued by uncomfortable and often disabling symptoms like bloating, cramps, diarrhoea, constipation, and pain.

Patients with IBS often were told to just get more fiber or take Metamucil, or were prescribed sedatives, anti-spasm drugs, or antidepressants. Most of commonly treatments don't work, because they don't address the underlying causes of why the digestion is not working. Emerging research has helped identify the underlying causes. If that lining breaks down — from stress, too many antibiotics or anti-inflammatory drugs like aspirin or Advil, steroids, intestinal infections, a low fiber, high-sugar diet, alcohol, and more – your immune system will be exposed to foreign particles from food and bacteria and other microbes. This will trigger and activate immune response, allergy, and will irritate the second brain (the enteric nervous system) creating havoc that leads to an irritable bowel, an irritable brain, and other system wide problems including allergy, arthritis, autoimmunity, mood disorders, and more.

The microbial ecosystem in the gut must be healthy for you to be healthy. When the gut bacteria are out of balance — when patient has too many pathogenic bacteria and not enough healthy bacteria — it makes them sick. We've got about 3 pounds of bacteria — 500 species — in the gut. In fact, there is more bacterial DNA in the body than there is human DNA! Among all that gut bacteria, there are good ones, bad ones, and very bad ones. If the bad ones take over — or if they move into areas that they shouldn't (like the small intestine which is normally sterile) — they can start fermenting the food we digest, particularly sugar or starchy foods.

This is called small bowel bacterial overgrowth, and it's a major cause of IBS. The major symptom it causes is bloating or a feeling of fullness after meals. Small bowel bacterial overgrowth can be diagnosed by a breath test, which measures gas production by the bacteria, or by a urine test that measures the by-products of the bacteria after they are absorbed into your system. Bacterial overgrowth is a real syndrome and was recently described in a review paper published in the Journal of the American Medical Association.(i) The condition can be treated. In fact, a major paper was recently published in the Annals of Internal Medicine that showed using a non-absorbed antibiotic called rifaximin for 10 days resulted in a dramatic improvement in bloating and overall symptoms of IBS by clearing out the overgrowth of bacteria. This medication is now under FDA review for approval as a new treatment for irritable bowel syndrome.

Migraine Medicines can ease migraines and other types of headaches, but people often use complementary and alternative treatments to get relief.

Stress is known to lead to some of the most common types of headaches, including migraines and tension headaches. So scientists have studied alternative treatments aimed at stress reduction, such as biofeedback and relaxation, and found that they work well for some people. Some people get relief from non-traditional headache treatments, including acupuncture, massage, herbs, and diets, but others don't. Migraine headaches are typically debilitating, and require a comprehensive approach for successful treatment. It is helpful to consider migraine headache as a symptom of an underlying imbalance, rather than simply a diagnosis. A holistic approach is a satisfying way to think about and treat migraine headache. Physicians trained in this approach will consider a broad array of features that may contribute to the experience of migraine headache, including disturbances within the following key areas:

- *Nutrition*
- *Digestion*
- *Detoxification*
- *Energy production*
- *Endocrine function*
- *Immune system function/inflammation*
- *Structural function*
- *Mind-body health*

Migraine headache is an excellent example of biologic uniqueness; the underlying factors participating in each individual's outcome may differ quite a bit from person to person. The journey of identifying and addressing these factors often results in an impressive improvement in frequency and intensity of the expression of migraine. Committed individuals will find the added benefit of better general health along the way. Patients will often request a more natural and self-directed approach to health care. The recommendations are typically very safe to implement, and are often welcomed by migraine sufferers. A practitioner with an integrative holistic focus will investigate an extensive array of predisposing factors to determine the underlying features most likely involved in a given individual's condition. In this way, we treat the individual, rather than his or her diagnosis, and we will generate a favourable impact upon his/her overall health in the process.

## Holy Basil and Rauwolfia Serpentina

Holy basil is a plant. It is originally from India and is used in Ayurvedic medicine as an "adaptogen" to counter life's stresses. It is considered a sacred plant by the Hindus and is often planted around Hindu shrines. The Hindu name for holy basil, Tulsi, means "the incomparable one." Medicine is made from the leaves, stems, and seeds. Holy basil is used for the common cold, influenza ("the flu"), H1N1 (swine) flu, diabetes, asthma, bronchitis, earache, headache, stomach upset, heart disease, fever, viral hepatitis, malaria, stress, and tuberculosis. It is also used for mercury poisoning, to promote longevity, as a mosquito repellent, and to counteract snake and scorpion bites.

Holy basil is applied to the skin for ringworm. In cooking, holy basil is often added to stir-fry dishes and spicy soups because of its peppery taste. Cookbooks sometimes call it "hot basil." Chemicals in holy basil are thought to decrease pain and swelling (inflammation). Other chemicals might lower blood sugar in people with diabetes. There is interest in using holy basil seed oil for cancer. Beginning research suggests that the oil can slow progression and improve survival rate in animals with certain types of cancer. Researchers think this benefit may be explained by the oil's ability to act as an antioxidant.

The Sanskrit name for Rauwolfia Serpentina/ Serpentine, Sarpagandha, means 'smelling like a snake', which refers to the herb's strong odor. The herb has a number of therapeutic benefits and has been used in Ayurvedic medicine for centuries.

Rauwolfia Serpentina is a central nervous system stimulant and also an anti-hypertensive. Its roots are known to treat intestinal disorders and also stimulate uterine contractions. A number of different species of the Rauwolfia plant are found all over India.

Reserpine is the principal constituent of Rauwolfia. It is credited with tranquilizing and anti-hypertensive properties. The chemical constituent ajmaline has anti-arrhythmic properties, which suppress abnormal rhythms of the heart. Rauwolfia is a key herb in the treatment of mild to moderate hypertension. It is also beneficial in the treatment of gastrointestinal disorders like cholera and colic. The herb is also helpful in treating gynecological disorders like leukorrhea.

## How to diagnose and differentiate Hysteria and Schizophrenia

Although the term "schizophrenia means "split mind," it does not refer to the splitting of the personality into several functioning personality subtypes as in dissociative identity disorder. Rather, the term was intended to convey a splitting of the normally integrated cognitive/behavioural/emotional functioning of the brain. For example, a person may suddenly become emotionally agitated even though there is no apparent objective reason for this change. Schizophrenia includes a variety of symptoms, not all of which will necessarily be present at any one time.

Hallucinations -- a hallmark of Schizophrenia. Usually, these take the form of hearing voices. These voices may be critical of the person, and in some cases may tell the person to do certain things. Visual Hallucinations are less common, but do occur in some cases.

Disordered Thought -- Thinking is irrational and disorganized.

Attentional Difficulties -- The person is easily distracted and has a difficult time focusing attention on one line of thought for long.

"Word Salad" -- In severe cases, the individual may exhibit such disordered thinking that sentences are almost completely disconnected, except perhaps by a chain of loose associations. Occasionally the person uses strange words ("neologisms") which seem to have a private meaning for the person and yet the person seems to believe that others know their meaning.

Delusions -- false beliefs that are firmly held regardless of evidence to the contrary. Paranoid delusions involve (a) delusions of grandeur -- an irrational belief that one is someone of elevated position or abilities, e.g., Christ; and (b) delusions of persecution -- an irrational belief that "they" are out to get you.

Catatonia -- the person "freezes" into a position of "waxy flexibility": you can reposition their arms etc. as if the person were a doll, and they will hold the new position (even a very uncomfortable one) for long periods of time. The person seems to be in a trance-like state, but upon emerging from the catatonia can report what had been happening.

Schizophrenia may be broken into two classes according to the rapidity of its development:

Reactive Schizophrenia
Symptoms develop over a period of days or weeks, usually in adulthood.
Good prognosis: the person is likely to recover from the disorder.
Process Schizophrenia
Symptoms develop gradually, over a period of months and years, usually beginning in the teens or early twenties.
Poor prognosis: the person is unlikely to recover from the disorder.

The causes of schizophrenia are unknown. Genetic factors may somewhat dispose one to develop the disorder, but even among identical twins, if one develops schizophrenia, the other has only about a 50-50 chance of developing it also, so there must be other precipitating factors. It is now known that there is some degree of brain deterioration associated with the disorder, at least in those diagnosed with "process" schizophrenia. A biochemical imbalance involving the neurotransmitter dopamine is implicated in the disorder, as drugs have proven effective in reducing the symptoms of schizophrenia tend to be those that reduce activity in the brain's dopamine systems.

Hysteria, in the colloquial use of the term, means ungovernable emotional excess. Generally, modern medical professionals have abandoned using the term "hysteria" to denote a diagnostic category, replacing it with more precisely defined categories, such as somatization disorder. In 1980, the American Psychiatric Association officially changed the diagnosis of "hysterical neurosis, conversion type" (the most extreme and effective type) to "conversion disorder". Current psychiatric terminology distinguishes two types of disorder that were previously labelled "hysteria": somatoform disorder and dissociative disorder. There are many cases of these disorders where nothing else can be diagnosed in the sufferers. The dissociative disorders in DSM-IV-TR include dissociative amnesia, dissociative fugue, dissociative identity disorder, depersonalization disorder, and dissociative disorder not otherwise specified. Somatoform disorders include conversion disorder, somatization disorder, pain disorder, hypochondriasis, and body dysmorphic disorder. In somatoform disorders, the patient exhibits physical symptoms, such as low back pain or limb paralysis, which have no apparent physical cause. Additionally, certain culture-bound syndromes – such as "ataques de nervios" ("attacks of nerves") identified in Hispanic populations, and popularized by Pedro Almodóvar's film Women on the Verge of a Nervous Breakdown – exemplify psychiatric phenomena which encompass both somatoform and dissociative symptoms, and have been linked to psychological trauma. Recent neuroscientific research is now beginning to show that there are characteristic patterns of brain activity associated with these states.[8] All these disorders are thought to be unconscious, not feigned and not intentional malingering.

Jungian psychologist Laurie Layton Schapira has explored the "Cassandra Complex" suffered by those traditionally diagnosed with hysteria. Basing her findings on clinical experience, she delineates three factors which constitute the Cassandra Complex in hysterics: (a) dysfunctional relationships, with social manifestations of rationality, order and reason, leading to (b) emotional or physical suffering, particularly in the form of somatic, often gynaecological complaints, and (c) sufferers being disbelieved or dismissed when attempting to relate the facticity of these experiences to others. The diagnosis of hysterical psychosis (HP) gained widespread recognition during the nineteenth century; but like the diagnosis of multiple personality disorder, the diagnosis of HP eventually faded from use. The concept of hysterical psychosis (HP) suffered a curious fate in the history of psychiatry. During the second half of the 19th century this disorder was well known and thoroughly studied, particularly in French psychiatry. In the early 20th century the diagnosis of hysteria, and of HP, fell into disuse. Patients formerly considered to suffer from HP were diagnosed schizophrenics or malingers. A few clinicians have attempted to reintroduce this diagnostic category, but it has not regained official recognition. (van der Hart, Witztum, & Friedman, 1993, p. 44)

The role of traumatically-induced dissociation in the etiology and clinical phenomenology of hysterical psychosis has been recognized by a growing number of contemporary authors, who differentiate this form of psychotic disorder from schizophrenia (Hirsch & Hollender, 1969; Hollender & Hirsch, 1964; Mallett & Gold, 1964; Spiegel & Fink, 1979; Steingard & Frankel, 1985; van der Hart & Spiegel, 1993;

van der Hart et al., 1993). Spiegel and Fink (1979) make the following distinctions between the diagnoses of schizophrenia and hysterical psychosis:

Our thesis is that the phenomena associated with the syndrome of hysterical psychosis may be simplified and understood best by reference to the profound hypnotic trance states of which such individuals are capable. From this point of view such hysterical symptoms as fugue states, amnesia, and hallucinations are understood as spontaneous, undisciplined trance states. Some individuals, in the face of dramatic stress within their family, at their job, or social pressure of other kinds may succumb to a psychotic form of communication which is different from schizophrenia in phenomenology, course, and prognosis. (p. 779) A number of additional authors concur with this distinction, emphasizing the role of high hypnotizability as an important factor in the differential diagnosis between hysterical psychosis and schizophrenia (Copeland & Kitching, 1937; Gross, 1980; Gruenewald, 1978; Hirsch & Hollender, 1969; Mallet & Gold, 1964; Steingard & Frankel, 1985; D. Spiegel & Greenleaf, 1992; H. Spiegel, 1991; van der Hart & D. Spiegel, 1993; van der Hart et al., 1993) . Steingard and Frankel (1985) also discuss the connection between high hypnotizability and dissociation in this clinical population: One important mechanism that we believe accounts for one type of transient or recurrent event of psychotic proportions is dissociation. Although the older literature on hypnosis (Janet, 1965) and its history (Ellenberger, 1970) and on dissociation (Nemiah, 1975; Frankel & Orne, 1976) have provided ample evidence of unusual behaviour in patients who dissociate easily and, at times, spontaneously, DSM-III failed to note the important coexistence of high hypnotizability and dissociative events. (p. 954) Also supporting this view are van der Hart et al. (1993) , who discuss their concerns regarding the confusion in diagnostic nomenclature pertaining to this clinical population: The Index of the DSM-III-R (American Psychiatric Association, 1987) contains HP, then refers readers to either Brief Reactive Psychosis or to Factitious Disorder with psychological symptoms .... In the case of reactive psychosis, we use the traditional nomenclature of HP in reviewing the literature and propose a new category of psychopathology - Reactive Dissociative Psychosis (RDP) . RDP integrates the classical features of HP with the most recent thinking on trauma-induced psychosis.... We believe that the essential characteristic for accurate diagnosis of RDP is not a short duration, hut a dissociative foundation....The dissociative foundation of RDP is a more meaningful explanatory principle than an hysterical or histrionic character as currently indicated in DSM-III-R. (pp. 44-45, 58) H. Spiegel (1991) expresses an additional concern:

"Without a careful differential diagnosis, hysterical psychosis and multiple personality disorder are often diagnosed as schizophrenia" (p. 164) . As an example, Murray (1993) offers a re-interpretation of the autobiographical account, I Never Promised You a Rose Garden (Greenberg, 1964/1981) . This classic tale traditionally has been presented as a case study on schizophrenia (Coleman & Broen, 1972). Murray's analysis questions the diagnosis of schizophrenia and focuses on the traumatic origins of the presenting symptomatology. Gainer (1992) similarly focuses on Greenberg' s account of childhood trauma, and identifies a number of the heroine 's presenting symptoms as characteristic examples of traumatic dissociation. I Never Promised You a Rose Garden tells the story of a troubled adolescent who is diagnosed with schizophrenia and is hospitalized at an inpatient facility for long-term psychiatric care. Author Joanne Greenberg, who originally published her book under the pseudonym of Hannah Green, has acknowledged the story's parallel with her own real life experiences as a patient under the care of Dr. Freida Fromm-Reichmann, at Chestnut Lodge during the 1940's and 1950's (Goodwin, 1993; Murray, 1993; Rubin, 1972). According to

Goodwin: " In those four years of analytic treatment, Fromm-Reichmann and the patient unrevealed the connections between these florid symptoms and the extensive medical trauma in early childhood that had schooled Joanne into escapes into fantasy" (Goodwin, 1990, p. 188). Fromm-Reichmann (1950) has described a case study which bears a strong resemblance to Greenberg's story, and which also illustrates Fromm-Reichmann ' s approach in treating dissociative symptoms with a traumatic origin. Asked if she could remember when being deceived had been linked up for the first time with the ether gun, she immediately recalled an operation which had been performed on her at the age of three. She had been told that it would not be she who would be operated on, but her doll. Ether was the anaesthetic used. The ether was administered suddenly while she was still expecting to see what was to be done to her doll. It was as if someone had shot ether at her. Before she was really under, things and people appeared tremendous, and the picture of the doctor who had operated on her had been retained in her memory ever since as that of a giant. Here was deception on the part of both of the patient's parents and of the doctor. It was connected with the sudden experience of the smell of ether imposed on her by a huge man. This, then was the actual experience which gave rise to the hallucinatory repetition of the experience which the patient underwent when she expected to be deceived by the psychiatrist. (Fromm-Reichmann, 1950, p. 174) Fromm-Reichmann conceptualizes in the following manner:

Descriptively speaking, hallucinations are perception without sensory foundation in the environment. Dynamically speaking, they owe their inception to the bursting-through into awareness of certain dissociated impulses which become so overwhelmingly strong that they cannot be retrieved in dissociation. (Fromm-Reichmann, 1950, p. 173)

Other related comments by Fromm-Reichmann have unmistakable relevance for contemporary psychotherapeutic work with the DID client: The psychoanalyst, as he works with a disturbed schizophrenic, is not only treating a child at different ages but also, and at the same time, an adult person of the chronological age in which he comes into treatment....Psychiatrists who are not sufficiently flexible may find it difficult to address themselves simultaneously to both sides of the schizophrenic personality. They may behave like rigid parents who refuse to realize that their children have grown up. The undesirable results of the psychiatrist's reluctance to communicate with the adult part in the patient's personality and his addressing himself only to the regressive parts in the patient have been discussed before.

If on the other hand, the psychotherapist addresses himself to the adult patient only, out of an erroneous identification with the patient, he renounces comprehension of and alertness to crucial parts of the schizophrenic psychopathology. (Fromm-Reichmann, 1948, p. 271)


## Menopause and how to treat it

Menopause, also known as the climacteric, is the time in most women's lives when menstrual periods stop permanently, and they are no longer able to bear children. Menopause typically occurs between

49 and 52 years of age. Medical professionals often define menopause as having occurred when a woman has not had any vaginal bleeding for a year. It may also be defined by a decrease in hormone production by the ovaries. In those who have had surgery to remove their uterus but they still have ovaries, menopause may be viewed to have occurred at the time of the surgery or when their hormone levels fell. Following the removal of the uterus, symptoms typically occur earlier, at an average of 45 years of age.

Before menopause, a woman's periods typically become irregular, which means that periods may be longer or shorter in duration or be lighter or heavier in the amount of flow. During this time, women often experience hot flashes; these typically last from 30 seconds to ten minutes and may be associated with shivering, sweating, and reddening of the skin. Hot flashes often stop occurring after a year or two. Other symptoms may include vaginal dryness, trouble sleeping, and mood changes. The severity of symptoms varies between women. While menopause is often thought to be linked to an increase in heart disease, this primarily occurs due to increasing age and does not have a direct relationship with menopause. In some women, problems that were present like endometriosis or painful periods will improve after menopause.

Menopause is usually a natural change. It can occur earlier in those who smoke tobacco. Other causes include surgery that removes both ovaries or some types of chemotherapy. At the physiological level, menopause happens because of a decrease in the ovaries' production of the hormones estrogen and progesterone. While typically not needed, a diagnosis of menopause can be confirmed by measuring hormone levels in the blood or urine. Menopause is the opposite of menarche, the time when a girl's periods start.

After menopause, hormone replacement therapy (HRT) is often prescribed to resupply the body with the hormones it no longer produces. There are a number of different treatment options to consider if you're suffering from symptoms of menopause.

HRT (also known as hormone therapy, menopausal hormone therapy, and estrogen replacement therapy) uses female hormones -- estrogen and progesterone -- to treat common symptoms of menopause and aging. Doctors can prescribe it during or after menopause. There are many types of estrogen therapy in many different forms -- pills, patches, suppositories, and more. The best type of hormone replacement therapy (HRT) depends on your health, your symptoms, personal preference, and what you need to get out of treatment.

Alternative and Natural Treatments
Supplements, herbs and botanicals like black cohosh, evening primrose oil, and flaxseed are thought to relieve menopausal symptoms.

Black Cohosh
Black cohosh, also known as black snakeroot or bugbane, is a medicinal root. It is used to treat women's hormone-related symptoms, including premenstrual syndrome (PMS), menstrual cramps, and menopausal symptoms.

Soy for Menopause Symptoms
Soy is high in isoflavones. Isoflavones are a type of phytoestrogen. Phytoestrogens are chemicals found in plants that work like estrogens.

Wild Yam and Progesterone Creams
Wild yam and progesterone creams are available without a prescription and are marketed for relieving perimenopausal symptoms caused by "estrogen dominance."
Nyasa is often performed before or during pujas (acts of reverence), at the hands of a seer or by the individual who is chanting or meditating. There are different types of nyasa practice. Some of the most common are:

## 5. Clinical Hypnotherapy

### Definition of hypnotic power and the concept of will power

Hypnosis is a state of human consciousness involving focused attention and reduced peripheral awareness and an enhanced capacity for response to suggestion. The term may also refer to an art, skill, or act of inducing hypnosis.

Theories explaining, what occurs during hypnosis fall into two groups. Altered state theories see hypnosis as an altered state of mind or trance, marked by a level of awareness different from the ordinary conscious state. In contrast, non-state theories see hypnosis as a form of imaginative role-enactment.

During hypnosis, a person is said to have heightened focus and concentration. The person can concentrate intensely on a specific thought or memory, while blocking out sources of distraction. Hypnotised subjects are said to show an increased response to suggestions. Hypnosis is usually induced by a procedure known as a hypnotic induction involving a series of preliminary instructions and suggestion. The use of hypnotism for therapeutic purposes is referred to as "hypnotherapy", while its use as a form of entertainment for an audience is known as "stage hypnosis". Stage hypnosis is often performed by mentalists practicing the art form of mentalism. Hypnotherapy or clinical hypnosis is a use of hypnosis in psychotherapy. It is used by licensed physicians, psychologists, and others.

Hypnotherapy is a helpful adjunct having additive effects when treating psychological disorders, such as these, along with scientifically proven cognitive therapies. Hypnotherapy should not be used for repairing or refreshing memory because hypnosis results in memory hardening, which increases the confidence in false memories.

Preliminary research has expressed brief hypnosis interventions as possibly being a useful tool for managing painful HIV-DSP because of its history of usefulness in pain management, its long-term effectiveness of brief interventions, the ability to teach self-hypnosis to patients, the cost-effectiveness of the intervention, and the advantage of using such an intervention as opposed to the use of pharmaceutical drugs.

Modern hypnotherapy has been used, with varying success, in a variety of forms, such as:

- *Charcot demonstrating hypnosis on a "hysterical" Salpêtrière patient, "Blanche" (Marie Wittmann), who is supported by Joseph Babiński*
- *Cognitive-behavioural hypnotherapy, or clinical hypnosis combined with elements of cognitive behavioural therapy*
- *Age regression hypnotherapy (or "hypnoanalysis")*
- *Ericksonian hypnotherapy*
- *Fears and phobias*
- *Addictions*
- *Habit control*
- *Pain management*
- *Psychotherapy*
- *Relaxation*
- *Skin disease*
- *Soothing anxious surgical patients*
- *Sports performance*
- *Weight loss*

In a January 2001 article in Psychology Today, Harvard psychologist Deirdre Barrett wrote:

A hypnotic trance is not therapeutic in and of itself, but specific suggestions and images fed to clients in a trance can profoundly alter their behaviour. As they rehearse the new ways they want to think and feel, they lay the groundwork for changes in their future actions...

Barrett described specific ways this is operationalized for habit change and amelioration of phobias. In her 1998 book of hypnotherapy case studies, she reviews the clinical research on hypnosis with dissociative disorders, smoking cessation, and insomnia, and describes successful treatments of these complaints. In a July 2001 article for Scientific American titled "The Truth and the Hype of Hypnosis", Michael Nash wrote that, "using hypnosis, scientists have temporarily created hallucinations, compulsions, certain types of memory loss, false memories, and delusions in the laboratory so that these phenomena can be studied in a controlled environment

'Will' is the ability to make conscious choice. We all have free will and make our own choices, even if these are to obey the commands of others. Flowers do not have will. Animals have a degree of will. Humans have more, simply because they are better at thinking and can make informed choices. When something can be done 'at will' means one can act at any time of choosing without hindrance. Greater will is needed when there are obstructions.

A person may be described as 'wilful' if they do not easily submit to the requests or commands of others. They do what they like, breaking rules and laws without concern for what others may think (other, perhaps, than to delight in the sense of control this brings).

Will is related to desire. If you do not want something very much, then the will to succeed is likely to be weak. This is reflected in the saying 'A faint heart never won a fair lady.' On the other hand if you have a strong desire, then you will be more likely to persist. Another saying is 'Where there's a will, there's a way.' Exertion of will as self-control may be viewed as a conflict of desires, for example where we both want to get angry and know that we should not. From a psychoanalytic position this looks like a conflict between id and superego. There is a scientific argument that our unconscious mind is actually in charge and that conscious thought is just the perceived surface of the total unconscious. Whether this is true or not, we still have what we call choice. The alternative is to be fatalistic and be blown by the winds of the world.

Willpower is the motivation to exercise will. A person with strong willpower will assert decisions even in the face of strong opposition or other contradictory indicators. A person with little willpower will give in easily. Getting what you want takes willpower, whether it means doing something or others doing things for you. To succeed, this means first you must know what you want. Then you must be determined to get it, even in the face of extreme difficulties. Will and power are closely related, as using will is exercising power. Powerful people often exercise what seems to be a strong will, although this often comes from the confidence that having power creates rather than directly from having the power. In a reversal, people who have strong a strong increase their power as a result.

Based upon the foresaid it is important to know, what suggestibility is. Suggestibility is the quality of being inclined to accept and act on the suggestions of others; where false but plausible information is given and one fills in the gaps in certain memories with false information when recalling a scenario or moment. Suggestibility uses cues to distort recollection after persistently being told something pertaining to a past event, one's memory of the event conforms to what they've been told. A person experiencing intense emotions tends to be more receptive to ideas and therefore more suggestible. Generally, suggestibility decreases as age increases. However, psychologists have found that individual levels of self-esteem and assertiveness can make some people more suggestible than others, which has resulted in the concept of a spectrum of suggestibility. Suggestibility is important in case of hypnosis.

## The ideal environment for practical hypnotism

Hypnosis should be conducted on a one-to-one basis in quiet and specifically designed offices. The hypnosis environment should be warmly decorated and furnished with comfortable reclining chairs ideally suited to help patients easily and comfortably to enter into hypnosis. It should be a quiet and friendly atmosphere without stress. Relaxing music may be helpful for patients to calm down. It is important to discuss the setting and patient status before treatment in a specific case history.

## Treatment of depression and anxiety neurosis by hypnotism

Hypnosis for depression can help address the underlying cause as well as help individuals find much more effective coping behaviours. It can also help people achieve a happier mood and decrease or dispel the pessimistic and negative thoughts that generally accompany depression. Hypnotherapy for this disorder will typically use a combination of suggestion and imagery to bring about positive changes in the unconscious processes of the depressed individual. People who undergo hypnosis for this disorder will often experience a new sense of freedom and a greater sense of control over their thoughts, their mood, and their life in general.

Since anxiety often goes hand in hand with depression, hypnosis can also be very beneficial because it helps reduce and often alleviate the anxious thoughts and feelings. Rather than remain stuck in the vicious cycle of painful thoughts and feelings of guilt, worthlessness, and hopelessness, hypnosis can help the person to develop a more positive outlook by using powerful self-suggestion. Rather than going through life reacting to difficult situations that would previously have felt overwhelming or hopeless, the individual learns how to respond effectively. The hypnotherapist may use positive affirmations and suggestions in a session once the individual has reached a state of deep relaxation. It is during this relaxed state that positive suggestions are very effective. For example, positive and present tense statements such as "I feel happy and optimistic, and am in control of my life", or "I am a worthwhile person who has much to offer others" may be used.

While not all depression is triggered by a traumatic or painful event, hypnosis can be a useful technique to help the individual learn new responses to painful triggers if indicated. It can also help the individual access distressful memories which were repressed yet contribute to the depressed mood. Hypnosis can bring those into conscious awareness and help the individual let go of painful or sad emotions associated with the event. Healthy and more positive associations which empower the individual can be learned to replace those which may have kept the individual depressed. In the future the individual will be less susceptible to similar events and will be able to respond to them more positively. While almost anyone can be put into a hypnotic trance, hypnosis will generally be more effective if the individual feels both at ease with and trusting of the hypnotherapist. Some people will experience positive effects from hypnosis sooner than others. Many factors will determine how quickly effects are experienced. Children respond more readily to hypnosis than adults, and will often experience significant improvement after just one or two sessions. Adults can vary greatly, depending on the severity of the depression, their personality makeup, their motivation for change and their openness to the hypnosis process among other things.

## The concept of Self- Hypnotism

Self-hypnosis, as the name suggests, is a way of creating the hypnotic trance state by ourselves, rather than relying on a hypnotist or hypnotherapist to do it for us. In every other respect, it's exactly the same as any other form of hypnosis. Indeed, some practitioners argue that all hypnosis is self-hypnosis, since it's a collaborative process that simply doesn't happen unless the subject agrees to participate in it.

In a formal hypnosis session, the hypnotist acts as a guide, leading the subject into a trance state by narrowing down the focus of attention and turning it inwards. This is developed with guided imagery and carefully constructed suggestions to achieve a desired end. In self-hypnosis you follow the same procedure, acting as your own guide into the trance state. This is, as far as we know, something that is unique to human beings - the ability of the human mind to contemplate and communicate with itself. There are many techniques for achieving self-hypnosis, and a simple one is outlined later in this article. But first of all, it's worth examining just why you should want to do this in the first place.

As with any form of hypnosis, the purpose of self-hypnosis is to establish communication with your own unconscious mind. It's a way of taking control of automatic behaviour and directing it in a more helpful way - to solve problems, access unconscious resources, learn more effectively, mentally rehearse a future event and so on. In cases of driving tests or sitting an exam, for instance, people may use self-hypnosis to vividly imagine feeling calm and in control whilst doing so. This will significantly improve the chances of success on the actual day. Another important aspect is the use of self-hypnosis to relax. This isn't to be underestimated. Regular deep relaxation promotes clear thinking, lowers blood pressure, boosts the immune system, encourages better sleep, makes you feel more energetic and generally reduces the toll that stress takes on your system. In short, it's a significant and easily obtained investment in mental and physical wellbeing, but one which modern life frequently seems to conspire against.

This is doubly concerning when we consider that our brains are supposed to relax in order to function properly. The cycle of the ultradian rhythm dictates that dominance switches from the left to the right brain hemisphere every ninety minutes, producing a feeling of daydream-like fuzziness for about fifteen minutes as the metaphorical, pattern matching right hemisphere assimilates everything that's happened over the previous hour and a half. Sadly, the demands of 21st century life mean that we often push on through this natural downtime, by charging ourselves up with caffeine or other stimulants, or through a sheer brute force act of concentration. This is like constantly driving a car at 80mph in low gear. Self-hypnosis is a way of cooling down and refuelling our mental engines by creating some of that natural downtime for ourselves. This allows the brain to do its housekeeping, switching off emotional arousals and flushing stress out of our system, keeping our mental and physical processes in good running order.

To practice self-hypnosis, we need to sit or lie quietly for a while without being disturbed. Self-hypnosis is different from meditation, in that the aim is not to clear the mind, but rather to direct it towards a purpose, so it's a good idea to have that purpose in mind before starting self-hypnosis. This might be mental rehearsal of a future event, or it might simply be to relax very deeply.

## Definition of neurosis and how to treat fears and phobias

Neurosis is a term generally used to describe a nonpsychotic mental illness which triggers feelings of distress and anxiety and impairs functioning. The word neurosis means "nerve disorder," and was first coined in the late eighteenth century by William Cullen, a Scottish physician. Cullen's concept of neurosis encompassed those nervous disorders and symptoms that do not have a clear organic cause. Sigmund Freud later used the term anxiety neurosis to describe mental illness or distress with extreme anxiety as a defining feature.

There is a difference of opinion over the clinical use of the term neurosis today. It is not generally used as a diagnostic category by American psychologists and psychiatrists any longer, and was removed from the American Psychiatric Association's Diagnostic and Statistical Manual of Mental Disorders in 1980 with the publication of the third edition (it last appeared as a diagnostic category in DSM-II). Some professionals use the term to describe anxious symptoms and associated behaviour, or to describe the range of mental illnesses outside of the psychotic disorders (such as schizophrenia, delusional disorder). Others, particularly psychoanalysts (psychiatrists and psychologists who follow a psychoanalytical model of treatment, as popularized by Freud and Carl Jung), use the term neurosis to describe the internal process itself (called an unconscious conflict) that triggers the anxiety characteristic.

The neurotic disorders are distinct from psychotic disorders in that the individual with neurotic symptoms has a firm grip on reality, and the psychotic patient does not. Before their reclassification, there were several major traditional categories of psychological neuroses, including: anxiety neurosis, depressive neurosis, obsessive-compulsive neurosis, somatization, posttraumatic stress disorder, and compensation neurosis-not a true neurosis, but a form of malingering, or feigning psychological symptoms for monetary or other personal gain.

Hypnosis has been shown to be an effective treatment for many individuals with phobias. A significant percentage of the population suffers from a phobia of one type or another. For some individuals it can be mildly distressing but manageable. For others it can be seriously debilitating. A phobia is an irrational fear of a particular stimulus. This stimulus can be a situation, a thing, or an activity. People with phobias will either go to great lengths to avoid whatever it is they fear, or they will tolerate it with considerable anxiety. For some people, a phobia can trigger panic attacks. In severe cases the phobia can end up literally controlling a person's life. Hypnotherapy works by accessing the underlying cause of the phobia and eliminating the person's conditioned response to the stimulus. When hypnosis is used to treat a phobia, the initial goal of the hypnotherapist is to discover the initial event from which the phobia developed. The cause is often a traumatic event which occurred at an earlier time in the person's life. Often the phobic individual does not remember this event. It may be a memory which has been repressed for many years. Repression is a protective mechanism our mind utilizes by keeping memory of the trauma out of our conscious mind until we are ready and able to deal with it.

In order to access this memory, the individual will first need to be in an extremely relaxed state. The hypnotherapist will use techniques in order to help the person become very relaxed and focused. This state of heightened relaxation and focus is referred to as the hypnotic trance. It is during this state that the unconscious can be accessed. While in this trance state a person is very receptive to suggestion, which is what opens the door to bringing about the desired change.

Also, it is during this trance state that unconscious memories can be unlocked and brought to conscious awareness. The hypnotherapist does this by taking the person back to the place and time where the distressing event occurred. Addressing this old memory consciously will enable the individual to better understand it as well as begin to see it in a way which is no longer threatening. When this is achieved, the phobia will generally disappear.  This process is referred to as hypnotic regression. While it can be very effective it can also be problematic. There is a lot of controversy around this technique because if not done correctly or ethically, false memories can also be created. This has led to many legal issues when hypnosis is used with witnesses or defendants in law suits and there is a question of false memories due to hypnosis.

In many cases, however, this is not an issue and the phobic response can be dealt with very effectively using hypnosis. The hypnotherapist can help the individual visualize himself facing the feared object or situation without experiencing any anxiety. The hypnotherapist can guide the person in creating new thoughts and responses regarding whatever it is he previously feared. The number of hypnosis sessions required for effectively dealing with phobias varies, and depends on several factors. These factors include how long the person has had the phobia, how severely the phobia affects him, the person's maturity, his personality structure, and how determined he is to be free from the phobia. In general, it will take approximately three or four hypnotherapy sessions.  However, in severe cases it can take more.

## Various levels of hypnosis

*Induction:* During induction, the hypnotherapist guides the client to narrowly focus his or her attention to the point that sensory impressions are blocked out. The client can then reach the state of complete relaxation necessary for hypnosis to occur. The hypnotherapist's office usually is quiet and dimly lit to create a relaxing atmosphere. The hypnotherapist chooses a particular method or combination of methods for induction based on the assessment of the client. An induction script may use different types of verbal and visual cues, including the following:

Use of authority: The hypnotherapist gives instructions in simple declarative sentences (e.g., "As I speak, you will relax.").

Guided visualization or imagery: The hypnotherapist suggests images or describes a scene for the patient (e.g., "Let your mind drift to a calm and peaceful place. See the wind blowing through the trees, the flowers in the meadow.").

Quiet music or rhythm: The hypnotherapist speaks in a steady, evenly paced rhythm without varying voice tone. Sometimes the therapist plays music in the background.

Repetition of words or sounds: The therapist repeats key words or sounds (e.g., "Breathe in deeply . . . ", "As you breathe in . . . ").

Emotional cues or probes: A hypnotherapy session may be used to gather more information about painful experiences or to help patients cope with difficult emotions. The therapist integrates the inquiries or instructions into the induction script (e.g., "You are in control and will choose to experience or ignore any suggestions during the session.").

Analogies, metaphors, and associative statements: The hypnotherapist uses comparisons to familiar experiences or images to help clients achieve physical relaxation (e.g., "Your legs are sinking into the couch, heavy as logs." "Feel your body, heavy and relaxed, being supported by the tree behind you, the ground beneath you.").

Clients do not always readily accept suggestions. The hypnotherapist is alert to any sign of negative reactions or abreactions that may occur during the induction. The hypnotherapist guides the client through these feelings or, if necessary, rewords the suggestion during a later session. An abreaction can present itself as a yawn, a frown, a scratch, or movement in the hand or foot. On occasion, clients might feel somewhat disoriented, or in rare instances, nauseous. Stopping the induction can usually relieve these effects, or they may disappear as the hypnotic state deepens. After the induction, some people report feeling different physical sensations (e.g. tingly, heavy, floating); others feel nothing unusual at all.

*Deepening:* Next, the hypnotherapist uses deepening techniques to enhance the hypnotic stage. These can include simply continuing the chosen induction, changing to another type, or talking directly to the client. There are three levels of hypnotic states:

- *Hypnoidal:* A light stage of hypnosis, characterized by fluttering eye movements
- *Cataleptic:* A deeper state, characterized by side-to-side eye movements
- *Somnambulistic:* The deepest state, characterized by the eyes rolling up

The somnambulistic level has three levels. The first two involve a kind of amnesia, that is, the client receives posthypnotic suggestions on a subconscious level and may not remember hearing them. The third level of somnambulism is so deep that a person in this state can undergo major surgery without anaesthesia.

For sessions focused on self-improvement or changing unwanted habits, the hypnoidal and cataleptic states are adequate; however, better results can be achieved if the client enters into the cataleptic state. Before moving on to the utilization stage, the hypnotherapist must be sure that the client is in a hypnotic state and ready to receive posthypnotic suggestions. There are several observable indicators of the hypnotic state:

- *Lack of body movement, stillness*
- *Pallid, waxen complexion*
- *Rapid eye movements, eyelid fluttering*
- *Redness around the eyes*
- *Relaxed posture, slumping*
- *Slowed breathing*
- *Swallowing, gulping*
- *Water or tears in the eyes*

*Utilization:* A posthypnotic suggestion is made during the utilization stage. The posthypnotic suggestion is a verbalized statement of the desired outcome. If taken in and acted upon, the suggestion affects behaviour after the client has emerged from hypnosis and returned to regular daily activities. The posthypnotic suggestion is the key to achieving the client's goal. As long as they are clear and specific in describing the goal, posthypnotic suggestions can be visual or auditory. Only positive suggestions based on the client's suggestibility effectively change behaviour. For example, the hypnotherapist might suggest that when a client finds him- or herself in a usually stressful situation, they will not desire a cigarette. An abreaction, such as a frown or shift in posture, may occur when the suggestion is made. Repeating the suggestion, rewording it, or choosing a different type of suggestion may help the client become more receptive. By repeating the suggestion to the client in each session, a new conditioned response may be achieved. The repeated chosen key words in the suggestion become associated with the desired outcome. If the client successfully receives the suggestion, he or she begins to formulate internal processes (emotions, visualizations, or dialogues), which help achieve the desired outcome. After the posthypnotic suggestion has been introduced and developed, the hypnotherapist leads the client into the termination stage.

*Termination:* Termination is the slow, gradual return to consciousness. Just prior to ending the hypnotic state, the hypnotherapist often repeats that the client is in control of his or her body and mind, and has been in control throughout the session. Several termination techniques may be used; the best known is counting backwards followed by the authoritative command "Wake up." The client opens their eyes and adjusts to the relaxed but aware state that follows hypnosis.

## How to give hypnotic suggestions and hypnotic initiations

Most hypnotic suggestions are very powerful when they affect posthypnotic. It's a powerful instruction that programs a person to act in a certain way, feel a certain feeling and/or do a specific behaviour ever after – for a prolonged period of time. This instruction is not consciously recognized because it's now part of the unconscious mind that runs their daily habits. To undo the suggestion, the person would generally have to once again enter a hypnotic state of trance and remove or change it.

Sometimes one Post Hypnotic Suggestion will actually be intensified by another suggestion "piggybacking" onto it at a later date – or may be superseded altogether by another suggestion that is emotionally stronger. Like any hypnotic process, Post Hypnotic Suggestions can be used to benefit, manipulate or to purposefully or accidentally do harm. There are many uses of Post Hypnotic Suggestions that you may not realize you're being exposed to in your day-to-day life. These could be unconsciously governing some of your thinking, behaviours and decisions.

We talk to our subject about the expectation for the session and what their perfect outcome would be. We have to make sure that Post Hypnotic Suggestion is very useful generally. For example, "You will continue to enjoy your life and find more and more happiness and opportunities coming your way." As with any hypnotic encounter, whether in casual conversation or therapy, you must follow the ABS Formula:

- Absorb the subject's full attention
- Bypass their critical factor
- Stimulate their unconscious mind

We use a hypnotic language, tone of voice and internal H+ (the intense desire that the person have a wonderfully successful experience with hypnosis) during our chitchat to gain rapport and put the person into a relaxed trance, (either with their eyes open or closed, depending on the situation). We access positive resources that the person has had in their past. Recollecting happy memories, successful times when they overcame an obstacle, successfully healed their body, felt adventurous and strong, conquered a fear or whatever state would come closest to accomplishing the outcome they want for the session. We explore the issue they've come to us for, and then link the positive resources we've elicited to the problem until the negative emotional loops have been dissolved. It is to test thoroughly that the problem is no longer accessible. When we're satisfied that the problem is no longer there, we can begin Post Hypnotic Suggestion(s). When we've gained subject's attention, it is to talk about something very positive for them – even if they don't have a problem to link it to. We can then give them a Post Hypnotic Suggestion. Give the Post Hypnotic Suggestions to them while they are still in a hypnotic trance in their most resourceful state after the problem is solved.

The following are commonly used hypnotic initiations with good results:

"Turn loose now, relax. Let a good, pleasant feeling come all across your body. Let every muscle and every nerve grow so loose and so limp and so relaxed. Arms limp now, just like a rag doll. That's good. Now, send a pleasant wave of relaxation over your entire body, from the top of your head to the tips of your toes. Just let every muscle and nerve grow loose and limp and relaxed. You are feeling more relaxed with each easy breath that you take. Droopy, drowsy and sleepy. So calm and so relaxed. You're relaxing more with each easy beat of your heart ... with each easy breath that you take ... with each sound that you hear"

"In a moment I'm going to relax you more completely. In a moment I'm going to begin counting backwards from 10 to 1. The moment I say the number 10 you will allow your eyelids to remain closed. The moment I say the number 10, you will, in your mind's eye, see yourself at the top of a small set of stairs. The moment I say the number 9, and each additional number, you will simply move down those stairs relaxing more completely. At the base of the stairs is a large feather bed, with a comfortable feather pillow. The moment I say the number one you will simply sink into that bed, resting your head on that feather pillow. Number 10, eyes closed at the top of those stairs. Ten ... Nine, relaxing and letting go. Nine ...Eight, sinking into a more comfortable, calm, peaceful position ...Seven ....Six ... going way down ...Five ... moving down those stairs, relaxing more completely. Four ... Three ... breathe in deeply ... Two ... On the next number, number one, simply sinking into that bed, becoming more calm, more peaceful, more relaxed ... One ... Sinking into that feather bed, let every muscle go limp and loose as you sink into a more calm, peaceful state of relaxation".

## How to treat neurosis and amnesia

Amnesia in hypnotic treatment is leads us to induce a regression (a phenomenon relevant to memory based upon age regression) of to come up with lost memories. In this phenomenon, it is suggested to subjects that they are turning back the calendar, and will relive an experience from some time and place in the past. The result can be a subjectively compelling return to childhood, as well as an objectively compelling display of childlike behaviour. But again, we have to distinguish between the imaginative experience constructed by hypnotic suggestion and the real thing: age-regressed subjects may genuinely believe that they are children again, and may behave in a childlike manner, but they do not grow smaller in the chair. For a long time there has been interest in what is happening psychologically to adults who have been regressed to childhood: to what extent do they return to mental states characteristic of childhood -- or, as Nash (1987, p. 42) put it, "What, if anything, is regressed about hypnotic age regression?".

There are at least three different facets of age regression which bear on questions of hypnosis and memory (Kihlstrom & Barnhardt, 1993). First is ablation: to what extent does an age-regressed person lose access to the fund of knowledge and repertoire of skills characteristic of his or her chronological age? This is really a question about both amnesia and agnosia, because the loss of access extends to semantic and procedural knowledge as well as episodic memory. The question of ablation is generally coupled to the conceptually distinct question of reinstatement: to what extent does an age-regressed adult return to archaic (to use a psychoanalytic concept), or at least chronologically earlier, modes of cognitive and emotional functioning? Ablation and reinstatement have been of considerable interest to developmental psychologists, especially those who embrace Piagetian ideas about qualitatively different stages in cognitive development. For example, what happens to pre-operational thought when a child moves into concrete operations? If one could somehow abolish conservation, and reinstate pre-operational modes of thought, that would tell us that these childlike modes of thinking may be preserved in the adult brain.

Of course, such a finding would also make it a lot easier to do developmental research -- if you can regress an adult to infancy, you do not have to cool your heels waiting for children to grow up. Something like this was actually attempted by Reiff and Scheerer (1959), with what appeared to be positive results, but a very careful replication by O'Connell, Shor, and Orne (1970) either failed to replicate their results or showed that they were artifacts of the demand characteristics of the testing situation. In a similar vein, studies employing a wide variety of experimental paradigms, including the Babinski reflex, various illusions which show developmental trends, and a host of tasks derived from the developmental theories of Heinz Werner and Jean Piaget (not to mention psychoanalysis), have yielded nothing by way of replicable evidence of ablation or reinstatement. Age-regressed adults may have the subjectively compelling experience of being children again, and they may appear to behave in a childlike manner, but what we see is an imaginative reconstruction of childhood -- not a reversion to the genuine article.

Despite the failure of age-regression to yield a faithful reproduction of childlike mental functioning, in principle the subjectively convincing experience of being a child again offers some promise for revivification. That is, in a manner analogous to state-dependent memory induced by changes in environmental context or emotional state, it might be that vividly imagining oneself as a child improves access to memories encoded during childhood. This is an interesting idea, but at present there is no convincing evidence for it. Only three published studies have actually attempted to corroborate the memories reported by age-regressed subjects. These all yielded results favorable to hypnosis, but they all suffer from serious methodological flaws that render their positive findings suspect (Kihlstrom & Barnhardt, 1993; Kihlstrom & Eich, 1994). There may be some memory enhancement produced by hypnotic age regression, but age regression is first and foremost a product of the imagination, and any accurate memory produced is likely to be blended with a great deal of false recall. The treatment of neurosis is equivalent to the treatment of phobias, as explained in Question 5 with nearly the same suggestions of freedom and calming down.

## Short notes on:   a)  Tratak  b) Nyasa dhyana

a)      According to Hathayog Pradipika, there are six types of hathayoga: dhauti, vasti, neti, nauli, tratak and kapalbhati. These are all yogic processes (shat karma) which apart from imparting physical and mental peace also provide spiritual power. The first four, i.e., dhauti, vasti, neti and nauli are related to purification of the body, while the last two, tratak and kapalbhati, are related to spiritual achievements. The flow of thoughts in our brain is an on-going process. Due to this, 80 per cent of our energy is wasted and our central nerve system loses its balance. But when we attain tratak sadhana, gradually we start experiencing peace of mind, and thereafter we start getting rid of unwanted thoughts. With this process we start gaining more and more energy. And a time comes when we are able to perform an unusual feat. But what is tratak sadhana? It is defined as focusing your attention with concentration on a point or on the flame of a lamp continuously, without blinking.

b)      In Hinduism, nyasa is a Tantric ritual that involves a series of touches in specific locations on the body. This is done by a "seer," or rishi, who chants a specific mantra to "place" it on a body part. It is thought that this ritual imparts the presence of a deity in the body, or makes the body of the individual more divine. In Sanksrit, nyasa means "placing" or "touching." In Tantric yoga or meditation, practitioners may lay hands on themselves or mentally "place" a mantra in specific locations on the body. Nyasa is often performed before or during pujas (acts of reverence), at the hands of a seer or by the individual who is chanting or meditating. There are different types of nyasa practice. Some of the most common are:

- *Rishi nyasa*
- *Kara nyasa*
- *Matrika nyasa*
- *Sadanga nyasa*

In some nyasa practices, a mantra from a book is considered ineffective. Instead, it is believed that the mantras should be produced by a rishi. The relaxation, meditation and visualization exercises (also called yoga nidra), that are used at the end of a yoga practice -- and, during which, practitioners "place" efforts of relaxation on specific body parts -- originally stem from mental nyasa rituals.

## 6. Anatomy

### The origin, insertion, nature supply and action of latissimus dorsi and gluteus maximus

The latissimus dorsi muscle, whose name means "broadest muscle of the back," is one of the widest muscles in the human body. Also known as the "lat," it is a very thin triangular muscle that is not used strenuously in common daily activities but is an important muscle in many exercises such as pull-ups, chin-ups, lat pulldowns, and swimming. The latissimus dorsi muscle has its origins along the lumbodorsal fascia of the lower back, arising from the inferior thoracic and lumbar vertebrae, sacrum, iliac crest, and the four most inferior ribs. From its many widespread origins, it runs obliquely, superiorly and laterally through the back and armpits to insert on the posterior side of the humerus of the upper arm. As the latissimus dorsi approaches its insertion point, the many muscular fibers from its many origins merge to a point, giving the muscle a triangular shape. The latissimus dorsi has several different functions, all of which involve movements of the arm. The primary function of the lat is the adduction of the arm, which is often used when performing a pull-up or chin-up or when pulling a heavy object down from a shelf above one's head. Another function of the lat is extension of the arm, as in swinging the arm toward the back. This motion is used when swinging the arms while walking as well as during rowing exercises. Finally, the latissimus dorsi medially rotates the arm, moving the front of the arm towards the body's midline. When performed with a bent elbow, medial rotation of the arm brings the hand towards the chest, like when folding the arms or touching the elbow on the opposite arm.

The gluteus maximus (also known collectively with the gluteus medius and minimus, as the gluteal muscles, and sometimes referred to informally as the "glutes") is the main extensor muscle of the hip. It is the largest and most superficial of the three gluteal muscles and makes up a large portion of the shape and appearance of each side of the hips. Its thick fleshy mass, in a quadrilateral shape, forms the prominence of the buttocks, the nates. Its large size is one of the most characteristic features of the muscular system in humans, connected as it is with the power of maintaining the trunk in the erect posture. Other primates have much flatter hips and can't sustain standing erectly. The muscle is remarkably coarse in function and structure, being made up of muscle fascicles lying parallel with one another, and collected together into larger bundles separated by fibrous septa.

# The bone and its classification with examples

A bone is a rigid organ that constitutes part of the vertebral skeleton. Bones support and protect the various organs of the body, produce red and white blood cells, store minerals and also enable mobility as well as support for the body. Bone tissue is a type of dense connective tissue. Bones come in a variety of shapes and sizes and have a complex internal and external structure. They are lightweight yet strong and hard, and serve multiple functions. Mineralized osseous tissue, or bone tissue, is of two types, cortical and cancellous, and gives a bone rigidity and a coral-like three-dimensional internal structure. Other types of tissue found in bones include marrow, endosteum, periosteum, nerves, blood vessels and cartilage.

Bone is an active tissue composed of different types of bone cells. Osteoblasts are involved in the creation and mineralisation of bone; osteocytes and osteoclasts are involved in the reabsorption of bone tissue. The mineralised matrix of bone tissue has an organic component mainly of collagen and an inorganic component of bone mineral made up of various salts.

In the human body at birth, there are over 270 bones, but many of these fuse together during development, leaving a total of 206 separate bones in the adult, not counting numerous small sesamoid bones. The largest bone in the body is the thigh-bone (femur) and the smallest is the stapes in the middle ear.

## The upper end of Femur in brief

The femur or thighbone, is the most proximal (closest to the hip joint) bone of the leg in tetrapod vertebrates capable of walking or jumping, such as most land mammals, birds, many reptiles such as lizards, and amphibians such as frogs. In vertebrates with four legs such as dogs and horses, the femur is found only in the hindlimbs. The head of the femur articulates with the acetabulum in the pelvic bone forming the hip joint, while the distal part of the femur articulates with the tibia and kneecap forming the knee joint. By most measures the femur is the strongest bone in the body. The femur is also the longest bone in the body. The upper or proximal extremity (close to the torso) contains the head, neck, the two trochanters and adjacent structures. The head of the femur, which articulates with the acetabulum of the pelvic bone, comprises two-thirds of a sphere. It has a small groove, or fovea, connected through the round ligament to the sides of the acetabular notch. The head of the femur is connected to the shaft through the neck or collum. The neck is 4–5 cm. long and the diameter is smallest front to back and compressed at its middle. The collum forms an angle with the shaft in about 130 degrees. This angle is highly variant. In the infant it is about 150 degrees and in old age reduced to 120 degrees on average. An abnormal increase in the angle is known as coxa valga and an abnormal reduction is called coxa vara. Both the head and neck of the femur is vastly embedded in the hip musculature and can't be directly palpated. In skinny people with the thigh laterally rotated, the head of the femur can be felt deep as a resistance profound (deep) for the femoral artery. The transition area between the head and neck is quite rough due to attachment of muscles and the hip joint capsule. Here the two trochanters, greater and lesser trochanter, are found. The greater trochanter is almost box-shaped and is the most lateral prominent of the femur. The highest point of the greater trochanter is located higher than the collum and reaches the midpoint of the hip joint. The greater trochanter can easily be felt. The trochanteric fossa is a deep depression bounded posteriorly by the intertrochanteric crest on medial surface of the greater trochanter. The lesser trochanter is a cone-shaped extension of the lowest part of the femur neck. The two trochanters are joined by the intertrochanteric crest on the back side and by the intertrochanteric line on the front. A slight ridge is sometimes seen commencing about the middle of the intertrochanteric crest, and reaching vertically downward for about 5 cm. along the back part of the body: it is called the linea quadrata (or quadrate line).

About the junction of the upper one-third and lower two-thirds on the intertrochanteric crest is the quadrate tubercle located. The size of the tubercle varies and it is not always located on the intertrochanteric crest and that also adjacent areas can be part of the quadrate tubercel, such as the posterior surface of the greater trochanter or the neck of the femur. In a small anatomical study it was shown that the epiphysial line passes directly through the quadrate tubercle.

## The ball and socket joint, the anatomy and movement of shoulder joint

Ball-and-socket joints are a special class of synovial joints that enjoy the highest freedom of motion in the body thanks to their unique structure. The shoulder and hip joints are the only ball-and-socket joints in the human body due to the need for great motion at the end of the body's limbs and the vast amount of musculature needed to move and support such flexible joints.

Two main components make up a ball-and-socket joint: a bone with a spherical head and a bone with a cup-like socket. In the shoulder joint, the spherical head of the humerus (upper arm bone) fits into the glenoid cavity of the scapula (shoulder blade). The glenoid cavity is a small and shallow cavity that permits the shoulder joint the greatest range of motion in the human body. A hyaline cartilage ring called the labrum surrounds the glenoid cavity to provide a flexible reinforcement to the joint, while muscles of the rotator cuff hold the humerus in place within the cavity.

The hip joint is somewhat less mobile than the shoulder, but is an overall stronger and more stable joint. The added stability of the hip joint is necessary to bear the weight of the body resting on the legs while performing actions such as standing, walking, and running. In the hip joint the rounded, almost spherical head of the femur (thigh bone) fits tightly into the acetabulum, a deep socket in the os coxa (hip bone). Many tough ligaments and the powerful hip muscles hold the head of the femur in place and resist some of the most powerful strains in the body. The depth of the acetabulum also prevents dislocations of the hip by limiting the movement of the femur within its socket.

Ball-and-socket joints are classified functionally as multiaxial joints because they can move bones along several axes. The muscles that surround the joints permit the humerus and femur to move away from the body's midline (abduction), toward the body's midline (adduction), forward (flexion), and backwards (extension). The humerus and femur can also move around the joint in a full circle (circumduction) as well as rotate both medially and laterally around their axis. Other parts of the body, such as the wrist and ankles, require at least two separate joints working together to achieve all of the movements of the ball-and-socket joints.

## Classification of the parts of brain with their importance

Brain Structures and their Functions

- *Cerebrum*
- *Cerebellum*
- *Limbic System*
- *Brain Stem*

The nervous system is your body's decision and communication center. The central nervous system (CNS) is made of the brain and the spinal cord and the peripheral nervous system (PNS) is made of nerves. Together they control every part of your daily life, from breathing and blinking to helping you memorize facts for a test. Nerves reach from your brain to your face, ears, eyes, nose, and spinal cord and from the spinal cord to the rest of your body. Sensory nerves gather information from the environment, send that info to the spinal cord, which then speed the message to the brain. The brain then makes sense of that message and fires off a response. Motor neurons deliver the instructions from the brain to the rest of your body. The spinal cord, made of a bundle of nerves running up and down the spine, is similar to a superhighway, speeding messages to and from the brain at every second.

The brain is made of three main parts: the forebrain, midbrain, and hindbrain. The forebrain consists of the cerebrum, thalamus, and hypothalamus (part of the limbic system). The midbrain consists of the tectum and tegmentum. The hindbrain is made of the cerebellum, pons and medulla. Often the midbrain, pons, and medulla are referred to together as the brainstem.

*The Cerebrum:* The cerebrum or cortex is the largest part of the human brain, associated with higher brain function such as thought and action. The cerebral cortex is divided into four sections, called "lobes": the frontal lobe, parietal lobe, occipital lobe, and temporal lobe. Here is a visual representation of the cortex:

Frontal Lobe- associated with reasoning, planning, parts of speech, movement, emotions, and problem solving

Parietal Lobe- associated with movement, orientation, recognition, perception of stimuli

Occipital Lobe- associated with visual processing

Temporal Lobe- associated with perception and recognition of auditory stimuli, memory, and speech

Note that the cerebral cortex is highly wrinkled. Essentially this makes the brain more efficient, because it can increase the surface area of the brain and the amount of neurons within it.
A deep furrow divides the cerebrum into two halves, known as the left and right hemispheres. The two hemispheres look mostly symmetrical yet it has been shown that each side functions slightly different than the other. Sometimes the right hemisphere is associated with creativity and the left hemisphere is associated with logic abilities. The corpus callosum is a bundle of axons which connects these two hemispheres.

Nerve cells make up the gray surface of the cerebrum which is a little thicker than your thumb. White nerve fibers underneath carry signals between the nerve cells and other parts of the brain and the body. The neocortex occupies the bulk of the cerebrum. This is a six-layered structure of the cerebral cortex which is only found in mammals. It is thought that the neocortex is a recently evolved structure, and is associated with "higher" information processing by more fully evolved animals (such as humans, primates, dolphins, etc).

*The Cerebellum:* The cerebellum, or "little brain", is similar to the cerebrum in that it has two hemispheres and has a highly folded surface or cortex. This structure is associated with regulation and coordination of movement, posture, and balance. The cerebellum is assumed to be much older than the cerebrum, evolutionarily. In other words, animals which scientists assume to have evolved prior to humans, for example reptiles, do have developed cerebellums. However, reptiles do not have neocortex.

*Limbic System:* The limbic system, often referred to as the "emotional brain", is found buried within the cerebrum. Like the cerebellum, evolutionarily the structure is rather old. This system contains the thalamus, hypothalamus, amygdala, and hippocampus.

*Brain Stem:* Underneath the limbic system is the brain stem. This structure is responsible for basic vital life functions such as breathing, heartbeat, and blood pressure. Scientists say that this is the "simplest" part of human brains because animals' entire brains, such as reptiles (who appear early on the evolutionary scale) resemble our brain stem. The brain stem is made of the midbrain, pons, and medulla.

## The structure and clinical importance of adrenal glands

The adrenal glands (also known as suprarenal glands) are endocrine glands that produce a variety of hormones including adrenaline and the steroids aldosterone and cortisol. They are found above the kidneys. Each gland has an outer cortex which produces steroid hormones and an inner medulla. The adrenal cortex itself is divided into three zones: zona glomerulosa, the zona fasciculata and the zona reticularis.

The adrenal cortex produces three main types of steroid hormones: mineralocorticoids, glucocorticoids, and androgens. Mineralocorticoids (such as aldosterone) produced in the zona glomerulosa help in the regulation of blood pressure and electrolyte balance. The glucocorticoids cortisol and corticosterone are synthesized in the zona fasciculata; their functions include the regulation of metabolism and immune system suppression. The innermost layer of the cortex, the zona reticularis, produces androgens that are converted to fully functional sex hormones in the gonads and other target organs. The production of steroid hormones is called steroidogenesis, and involves a number of reactions and processes that take place in cortical cells. The medulla produces the catecholamines adrenaline and noradrenaline, which function to produce a rapid response throughout the body in stress situations.

A number of endocrine diseases involve dysfunctions of the adrenal gland. Overproduction of cortisol leads to Cushing's syndrome, whereas insufficient production is associated with Addison's disease. Congenital adrenal hyperplasia is a genetic disease produced by dysregulation of endocrine control mechanisms. A variety of tumors can arise from adrenal tissue and are commonly found in medical imaging when searching for other diseases. The adrenal glands are located on both sides of the body in the retroperitoneum, above and slightly medial to the kidneys. In humans, the right adrenal gland is pyramidal in shape, whereas the left is semilunar and somewhat larger.[8] The glands are usually about 5x3 cm in size, and their combined weight in an adult human ranges from 7 to 10 grams. The glands are yellowish in colour.

The adrenal glands are surrounded by a fatty capsule and lie within the renal fascia, which also surrounds the kidneys. A weak wall of connective tissue separates the glands from the kidneys. The adrenal glands are directly below the diaphragm, and are attached to the crura of the diaphragm by the renal fascia. Each adrenal gland has two distinct parts, each with a unique function, the outer adrenal cortex and the inner medulla, both of which produce hormones.

## The pericardium with its anatomy of atrium and ventricles

The heart is a muscular organ in humans and other animals, which pumps blood through the blood vessels of the circulatory system. Blood provides the body with oxygen and nutrients, as well as assists in the removal of metabolic wastes. The heart is located in the middle compartment of the chest.

In humans, the heart is divided into four chambers: upper left and right atria; and lower left and right ventricles. Commonly the right atrium and ventricle are referred together as the right heart and their left counterparts as the left heart. In a healthy heart blood flows one way through the heart due to heart valves, which prevent backflow. The heart is enclosed in a protective sac, the pericardium, which also contains a small amount of fluid. The wall of the heart is made up of three layers: epicardium, myocardium, and endocardium.

The heart is a muscular organ that pumps blood throughout the body, with a rhythm determined by a group of pacemaking cells in the sinoatrial node. These generate a current that causes contraction of the heart, traveling through the atrioventricular node and along the conduction system of the heart. The heart receives blood low in oxygen from the systemic circulation, which enters the right atrium from the superior and inferior venae cavae and passes to the right ventricle. From here it is pumped into the pulmonary circulation, through the lungs where it receives oxygen and gives off carbon dioxide. Oxygenated blood then returns to the left atrium, passes through the left ventricle and is pumped out through the aorta to the systemic circulation–where the oxygen is used and metabolized to carbon dioxide. The heart beats at a resting rate close to 72 beats per minute.[9] Exercise temporarily increases the rate, but lowers resting heart rate in the long term, and is good for heart health.

Cardiovascular diseases (CVD) are the most common cause of death globally as of 2008, accounting for 30% of deaths. Of these more than three quarters are a result of coronary artery disease and stroke. Risk factors include: smoking, being overweight, little exercise, high cholesterol, high blood pressure, and poorly controlled diabetes, among others. Cardiovascular diseases frequently have no symptoms or may cause chest pain or shortness of breath. Diagnosis of heart disease is often done by the taking of a medical history, listening to the heart-sounds by auscultation, ECG, and ultrasound.

## The anatomical consideration of Mediastinum and Thoracic Cavity

The mediastinum (from Medieval Latin Mediastinus, "midway" is the central compartment of the thoracic cavity surrounded by loose connective tissue, as an undelineated region that contains a group of structures within the thorax. The mediastinum contains the heart and its vessels, the esophagus, trachea, phrenic and cardiac nerves, the thoracic duct, thymus and lymph nodes of the central chest. The mediastinum lies within the thorax and is enclosed on the right and left by pleurae. It is surrounded by the chest wall in front, the lungs to the sides and the spine at the back. It extends from the sternum in front to the vertebral column behind, and contains all the organs of the thorax except the lungs. It is continuous with the loose connective tissue of the neck.

The mediastinum can be divided into an upper (or superior) and lower (or inferior) part:

The superior mediastinum starts at the superior thoracic aperture and ends at the thoracic plane.
The thoracic plane separates the superior and inferior mediastinum. It is a plane at the level of the sternal angle , and the intervertebral disc of T4-T5.
The inferior mediastinum from this level to the diaphragm. This lower part is subdivided into three regions, all relative to the pericardium - the anterior mediastinum being in front of the pericardium, the middle mediastinum contains the pericardium and its contents, and the posterior mediastinum being behind the pericardium.

Anatomists, surgeons, and clinical radiologists compartmentalize the mediastinum differently. For instance, in the radiological scheme of Felson, there are only three compartments (anterior, middle, and posterior), and the heart is part of the anterior mediastinum.

The mediastinum is frequently the site of involvement of various tumors:
Anterior mediastinum: substernal thyroid goiters, lymphoma, thymoma, and teratoma.
Middle mediastinum: lymphadenopathy, metastatic disease such as from small cell carcinoma from the lung.
Posterior mediastinum: Neurogenic tumors, either from the nerve sheath (mostly benign) or elsewhere (mostly malignant).
Mediastinitis is inflammation of the tissues in the mediastinum, usually bacterial and due to rupture of organs in the mediastinum. As the infection can progress very quickly, this is a serious condition.

Pneumomediastinum is the presence of air in the mediastinum, which in some cases can lead to pneumothorax, pneumoperitoneum, and pneumopericardium if left untreated. However, that does not always occur and sometimes those conditions are actually the cause, not the result, of pneumomediastinum. These conditions frequently accompany Boerhaave's syndrome, or spontaneous esophageal rupture.

There are many diseases that can present with a widened mediastinum (usually found via a chest x-ray). The most common ones are aortic unfolding, traumatic aortic rupture, thoracic aortic aneurysm, and traumatic thoracic vertebral fracture. A widened mediastinum is a classic but rare hallmark sign of anthrax infection.

## The surface anatomy of inguinal canal with inguinal ring and urogenital diaphragm

The inguinal canal is a passage in the anterior abdominal wall that in men conveys the spermatic cord and in women the round ligament of uterus. The inguinal canal is larger and more prominent in men. There is one inguinal canal on each side of the midline. The inguinal canal is situated just above the medial half of the inguinal ligament. In both sexes the canal transmits the ilioinguinal nerve. The canal is approximately 3.75 to 4 cm long.[citation needed], angled anteroinferiorly and medially.

A first-order approximation is to visualize the canal as a cylinder. The structures which pass through the canal differ between males and females:

In males: the spermatic cord and its coverings + the ilioinguinal nerve.
In females: the round ligament of the uterus + the ilioinguinal nerve.
The classic description of the contents of spermatic cord in the male are:

3 arteries: artery to vas deferens (or ductus deferens), testicular artery, cremasteric artery;
3 fascial layers: external spermatic, cremasteric, and internal spermatic fascia;
3 other structures: pampiniform plexus, vas deferens (ductus deferens), testicular lymphatics;
3 nerves: genital branch of the genitofemoral nerve (L1/2), sympathetic and visceral afferent fibres, ilioinguinal nerve (N.B. outside spermatic cord but travels next to it)
Note that the ilioinguinal nerve passes through the superficial ring to descend into the scrotum, but does not formally run through the canal.

## Short notes on: a) Circle of Willis and b) Inferior Surface of Liver

a) The circle of Willis (circulus arteriosus cerebri) is an anastomotic system of arteries that sits at the base of the brain. The "circle" was named after Thomas Willis by his student Richard Lower. Willis was the author of Cerebri Anatome, a book that described and depicted this vascular ring.

Although such a vascular ring had been described earlier, the name Willis has been eponymously propagated.

The circle of Willis encircles the stalk of the pituitary gland and provides important communications between the blood supply of the forebrain and hindbrain (ie, between the internal carotid and vertebrobasilar systems following obliteration of primitive embryonic connections). A complete circle of Willis is present in most individuals, although a well-developed communication between each of its parts is identified in less than half of the population.

The circle of Willis is formed when the internal carotid artery (ICA) enters the cranial cavity bilaterally and divides into the anterior cerebral artery (ACA) and middle cerebral artery (MCA). The anterior cerebral arteries are then united by an anterior communicating (ACOM) artery. These connections form the anterior half (anterior circulation) of the circle of Willis. Posteriorly, the basilar artery, formed by the left and right vertebral arteries, branches into a left and right posterior cerebral artery (PCA), forming the posterior circulation. The PCAs complete the circle of Willis by joining the internal carotid system anteriorly via the posterior communicating (PCOM) arteries.

b) The liver is a vital organ of vertebrates and some other animals. In the human, it is located in the upper right quadrant of the abdomen, below the diaphragm. The liver has a wide range of functions, including detoxification of various metabolites, protein synthesis, and the production of biochemicals necessary for digestion.

The liver is a gland and plays a major role in metabolism with numerous functions in the human body, including regulation of glycogen storage, decomposition of red blood cells, plasma protein synthesis, hormone production, and detoxification. It is an accessory digestive gland and produces bile, an alkaline compound which aids in digestion via the emulsification of lipids. The gallbladder, a small pouch that sits just under the liver, stores bile produced by the liver. The liver's highly specialized tissue consisting of mostly hepatocytes regulates a wide variety of high-volume biochemical reactions, including the synthesis and breakdown of small and complex molecules, many of which are necessary for normal vital functions. Estimates regarding the organ's total number of functions vary, but textbooks generally cite it being around 500. Terminology related to the liver often starts in hepat- from the Greek word for liver.

There is currently no way to compensate for the absence of liver function in the long term, although liver dialysis techniques can be used in the short term. Artificial livers are yet to be developed to promote long term replacement in the absence of the liver. As of now, liver transplantation is the only option for complete liver failure.
On the diaphragmatic surface, apart from a large triangular bare area where it connects to the diaphragm, the liver is covered by a thin double-layered membrane, the peritoneum, that help reduces friction against other organs. This surface covers the convex shape of the two lobes where it accommodates the shape of the diaphragm. The peritoneum folds back on itself to form the

falciform ligament and the right and left triangular ligaments. These peritoneal ligaments are not related to the anatomic ligaments in joints, and the right and left triangular ligaments have no known functional importance, though they serve as surface landmarks. The falciform ligament functions to attach the liver to the posterior portion of the anterior body wall. The visceral surface or inferior surface, is uneven and concave. It is covered in peritoneum apart from where it attaches the gallbladder and the porta hepatis.

## 7. *Physiology*

### Definition of a human cell with diagram

The cell (from Latin cella, meaning "small room") is the basic structural, functional, and biological unit of all known living organisms. A cell is the smallest unit of life that can replicate independently, and cells are often called the "building blocks of life". The study of cells is called cell biology.

Cells consist of cytoplasm enclosed within a membrane, which contains many biomolecules such as proteins and nucleic acids. Organisms can be classified as unicellular (consisting of a single cell; including bacteria) or multicellular (including plants and animals). While the number of cells in plants and animals varies from species to species, humans contain more than 10 trillion (1013) cells.

The cell was discovered by Robert Hooke in 1665, who named the biological unit for its resemblance to cells inhabited by Christian monks in a monastery. Cell theory, first developed in 1839 by Matthias Jakob Schleiden and Theodor Schwann, states that all organisms are composed of one or more cells, that cells are the fundamental unit of structure and function in all living organisms, that all cells come from preexisting cells, and that all cells contain the hereditary information necessary for regulating cell functions and for transmitting information to the next generation of cells. Cells emerged on Earth at least 3.5 billion years ago. Each cell contains all of the genetic information necessary to manufacture a human being. This information is encoded within the cell nucleus in 6 billion subunits of DNA called base pairs. These base pairs are packaged in 23 pairs of chromosomes, with 1 chromosome in each pair coming from each parent. Each of the 46 human chromosomes contains the DNA for thousands of individual genes.

Diagram:

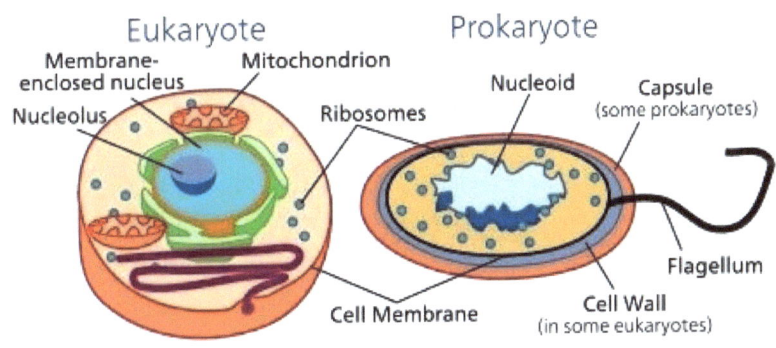

## The properties of muscles and the Cross Bridge Theory

Muscle cells, also known as muscle fibers or myocytes, are the fundamental units of the muscles. Humans have three types of muscle: skeletal, smooth and cardiac. The skeletal muscles are under conscious control, while the smooth muscle -- found in the walls of the blood vessels and hollow organs -- and cardiac muscle are not. All muscle cells share four primary properties that distinguish them from other cells.

### Excitability

For a muscle to contract and do work, its cells must be stimulated, most often by the nerves supplying them. Nervous impulses cause the release of the neurotransmitter acetylcholine at the nerve-muscle junction, and the acetylcholine activates receptors on the surface of the muscle cell. This results in an influx of positively charged sodium ions into the muscle cell and a depolarization of the muscle cell membrane, which in the resting state is quite negatively charged. If the membrane becomes sufficiently depolarized, an action potential results; the muscle cell is then "excited" from an electrochemical standpoint.

### Contractility

In the case of skeletal muscles, muscle cells contract when stimulated by neural input; smooth and cardiac muscles do not require this input. When a muscle cell is excited, the impulse travels along various membranes of the cell to its interior, where it leads to the opening of calcium channels. Calcium ions flow toward and bind to a protein molecule called troponin, leading to sequential changes in shape and position of the associated proteins tropomyosin, myosin and actin. The upshot is that myosin binds to small strands within the cell called myofilaments and pulls them along, causing the cell to shorten, or contract. Since this is going on simultaneously and in a coordinated fashion in many thousands of myocytes at the same time, the muscle as a whole contracts.

### Extensibility

Most of your body's cells lack the capacity to stretch; attempting to do so only damages or destroys them. Your long, cylindrical muscle cells, however, are a different story. Muscle cells contract, and in order for them to retain this ability, they must accordingly possess extensibility, or the capacity to lengthen. Your muscle cells can be stretched to about three times their contracted length without rupturing. This is important because in a lot of coordinated movements, so-called antagonistic muscles operate such that one is lengthening while the other is contracting. For example, when you run, the hamstring in the back of your thigh contracts while your quadriceps are extended and conversely.

### Elasticity

When something is described as elastic, this is simply a statement that it can be stretched or contracted by some amount above or below its resting or default length without damaging it, and that it will return to this resting length once the stimulus for stretching or contraction is removed. Your muscles require the property of elastic recoil for them to be able to do their jobs. If, say, your biceps muscles failed to recoil to their resting length after being stretched during a series of curling exercises, they would become slack, and slack muscles with no tension are unable to generate any force and are therefore useless as levers.

The Sliding Filament Theory or Cross Bridge Theory: At a very basic level each muscle fibre is made up of smaller fibres called myofibrils. These contain even smaller structures called actin and myosin filaments. These filaments slide in and out between each other to form a muscle contractions, hence called the sliding filament theory.

The myofibril called a sarcomere is the smallest unit of skeletal muscle that can contract. Sarcomeres repeat themselves over and over along the length of the myofibril.

All of the following structures are involved:

*Myofibril:* A cylindrical organelle running the length of the muscle fibre, containing Actin and Myosin filaments.
*Sarcomere:* The functional unit of the Myofibril, divided into I, A and H bands.
*Actin:* A thin, contractile protein filament, containing 'active' or 'binding' sites.
*Myosin:* A thick, contractile protein filament, with protusions known as Myosin Heads.
*Tropomyosin:* An actin-binding protein which regulates muscle contraction.
*Troponin:* A complex of three proteins, attached to Tropomyosin.
Here is what happens in detail. The process of a muscle contracting can be divided into 5 sections:

A nervous impulse arrives at the neuromuscular junction, which causes a release of a chemical called Acetylcholine. The presence of Acetylcholine causes the depolarisation of the motor end plate which travels throughout the muscle by the transverse tubules, causing Calcium (Ca+) to be released from the sarcoplasmic reticulum.
In the presence of high concentrations of Ca+, the Ca+ binds to Troponin, changing its shape and so moving Tropomyosin from the active site of the Actin. The Myosin filaments can now attach to the Actin, forming a cross-bridge.
The breakdown of ATP releases energy which enables the Myosin to pull the Actin filaments inwards and so shortening the muscle. This occurs along the entire length of every myofibril in the muscle cell.
The Myosin detaches from the Actin and the cross-bridge is broken when an ATP molecule binds to the Myosin head. When the ATP is then broken down the Myosin head can again attach to an Actin binding site further along the Actin filament and repeat the 'power stroke'. This repeated pulling of the Actin over the myosin is often known as the ratchet mechanism.
This process of muscular contraction can last for as long as there is adequate ATP and Ca+ stores. Once the impulse stops the Ca+ is pumped back to the Sarcoplasmic Reticulum and the Actin returns to its resting position causing the muscle to lengthen and relax.
It is important to realise that a single power stroke results in only a shortening of approximately 1% of the entire muscle. Therefore to achieve an overall shortening of up to 35% the whole process must be repeated many times. It is thought that whilst half of the cross-bridges are active in pulling the Actin over the Myosin, the other half are looking for their next binding site.

## The formation and importance of Cervical Plexus

The cervical plexus is a plexus of the anterior rami of the first four cervical spinal nerves which are located from C1 to C4 cervical segment in the neck. They are located laterally to the transverse processes between prevertebral muscles from the medial side and vertebral (m. scalenus, m. levator scapulae, m. splenius cervicis) from lateral side. There is anastomosis with accessory nerve, hypoglossal nerve and sympathetic trunk.

It is located in the neck, deep to sternocleidomastoid. Nerves formed from the cervical plexus innervate the back of the head, as well as some neck muscles. The branches of the cervical plexus emerge from the posterior triangle at the nerve point, a point which lies midway on the posterior border of the sternocleidomastoid.

The cervical plexus has two types of branches: cutaneous and muscular.

Cutaneous (4 branches):
Great auricular nerve - innervates skin near concha auricle (outer ear) and external acoustic meatus (ear canal) (C2&C3)
Transverse cervical nerve - innervates anterior region of neck (C2&C3)
Lesser occipital - innervates the skin and the scalp posterosuperior to the auricle (C2)
Supraclavicular nerves - innervate the skin above and below the clavicle (C3,C4)
Muscular
Ansa cervicalis (loop formed from C1-C3), etc. (geniohyoid (C1 only), thyrohyoid (C1 only), sternothyroid, sternohyoid, omohyoid)
Phrenic (C3-C5 (primarily C4))-innervates diaphragm and the pericardium
Segmental branches (C1-C4)- innervates anterior and middle scalenes
Additionally there are two branches formed by the posterior roots of spinal nerves:

Preauricular nerve (from the posterior roots of C2–C3)
Postauricular nerve (from the posterior roots of C3–C4)

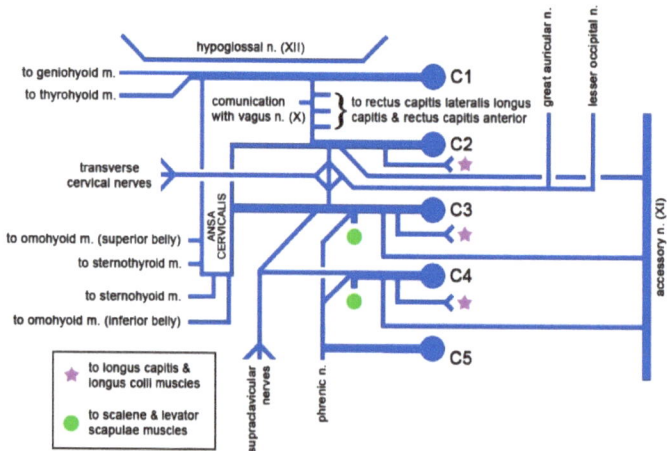

## The Menstruation and Menstruation Phases

The menstrual cycle is the series of changes the body goes through to prepare for a possible pregnancy. About once a month, the uterus grows a new, thickened lining (endometrium) that can hold a fertilized egg. When there is no fertilized egg to start a pregnancy, the uterus then sheds its lining. This is the monthly menstrual bleeding (also called menstruation or menstrual period) that you have from your early teen years until your menstrual periods end around age 50 (menopause).

The menstrual cycle is measured from the first day of menstrual bleeding, Day 1, up to Day 1 of your next menstrual bleeding. Although 28 days is the average cycle length, it is normal to have a cycle that is shorter or longer.

A teen's cycles may be long (up to 45 days), growing shorter over several years.
Between ages 25 and 35, most women's cycles are regular, generally lasting 21 to 35 days.
Around ages 40 to 42, cycles tend to be the shortest and most regular. This is followed by 8 to 10 years of longer, less predictable cycles until menopause

On Day 1 of your cycle, the thickened lining (endometrium) of the uterus begins to shed. We know this as menstrual bleeding from the vagina. A normal menstrual period can last 4 to 6 days.

Most of the menstrual blood loss happens during the first 3 days. This is also when you might have cramping pain in your pelvis, legs, and back. Cramps can range from mild to severe. The cramping is your uterus contracting, helping the endometrium shed. In general, any premenstrual symptoms that you've felt before your period will go away during these first days of the cycle.

*Follicular Phase*
During the follicular phase, an egg follicle on an ovary gets ready to release an egg. Usually, one egg is released each cycle. This process can be short or long and plays the biggest role in how long the cycle is. At the same time, the uterus starts growing a new endometrium to prepare for pregnancy.

The last 5 days of the follicular phase, plus ovulation day, are your fertile window. This is when you are most likely to become pregnant if you have sex without using birth control.

*Luteal (premenstrual) Phase*

This phase starts on ovulation day, the day the egg is released from the egg follicle on the ovary. It can happen any time from Day 7 to Day 22 of a normal menstrual cycle. During ovulation, some women have less than a day of red spotting or lower pelvic pain or discomfort. These signs of ovulation are normal.

If the egg is fertilized by sperm and then implants in (attaches to) the endometrium, a pregnancy begins. (This pregnancy is dated from Day 1 of this menstrual cycle.) If the egg is not fertilized or does not implant, the endometrium begins to break down.

After the teen years and before perimenopause in your 40s, the luteal phase is very predictable. It normally lasts 13 to 15 days, from ovulation until menstrual bleeding starts a new cycle. This 2-week period is also called the "premenstrual" period.

Many women have premenstrual symptoms during all or part of the luteal phase. They may feel tense, angry, or emotional, gain water weight and feel bloated or may have tender breasts or acne. A day or more before the period, women may start to have pain (cramps) in lower abdomen, back, or legs. It is normal to have less energy at this time. Some women also have headaches, diarrhea or constipation, nausea, dizziness, or fainting.

## The structure and function of the kidney

The kidneys are bean-shaped organs that serve several essential regulatory roles in vertebrates. Their main function is to regulate the balance of electrolytes in the blood, along with maintaining pH homeostasis. They also remove excess organic molecules from the blood, and it is by this action that their best-known function is performed: the removal of waste products of metabolism. Kidneys are essential to the urinary system and also serve homeostatic functions such as the regulation of electrolytes (including salts), maintenance of acid–base balance, maintenance of fluid balance, and regulation of blood pressure (via the salt and water balance). They serve the body as a natural filter of the blood, and remove water-soluble wastes which are diverted to the bladder. In producing urine, the kidneys excrete nitrogenous wastes such as urea and ammonium. They are also responsible for the reabsorption of water, glucose, and amino acids. The kidneys also produce hormones including calcitriol and erythropoietin. An important enzyme, renin, is also produced in the kidneys; it acts in negative feedback.

Located at the rear of the abdominal cavity in the retroperitoneal space, the kidneys receive blood from the paired renal arteries, and drain into the paired renal veins. Each kidney excretes urine into a ureter which empties into the bladder.

Renal physiology is the study of kidney function, while nephrology is the medical specialty concerned with kidney diseases. Diseases of the kidney are diverse, but individuals with kidney disease frequently display characteristic clinical features. Common clinical conditions involving the kidney include the nephritic and nephrotic syndromes, renal cysts, acute kidney injury, chronic kidney disease, urinary tract infection, nephrolithiasis, and urinary tract obstruction. Various cancers of the kidney exist. The most common adult renal cancer is renal cell carcinoma. Cancers, cysts, and some other renal conditions can be managed with removal of the kidney. This is known as nephrectomy. When renal function, measured by the glomerular filtration rate, is persistently poor, dialysis and kidney transplantation may be treatment options. Although they are not normally harmful, kidney stones can be extremely painful.

In humans, the kidneys are located high in the abdominal cavity, one on each side of the spine, and lie in a retroperitoneal position at a slightly oblique angle. The asymmetry within the abdominal cavity, caused by the position of the liver, typically results in the right kidney being slightly lower and smaller than the left, and being placed slightly more to the middle than the left kidney. The left kidney is approximately at the vertebral level T12 to L3, and the right is slightly lower. The right kidney sits just below the diaphragm and posterior to the liver. The left sits below the diaphragm and posterior to the spleen. On top of each kidney is an adrenal gland. The upper parts of the kidneys are partially protected by the 11th and 12th ribs. Each kidney, with its adrenal gland is surrounded by two layers of fat: the perinephric fat present between renal fascia and renal capsule and paranephric fat superior to the renal fascia.

The kidney has a bean-shaped structure having a convex and a concave border. A recessed area on the concave border is the renal hilum, where the renal artery enters the kidney and the renal vein and ureter leave. The kidney is surrounded by tough fibrous tissue, the renal capsule, which is itself surrounded by perirenal fat (adipose capsule), renal fascia, and pararenal fat (paranephric body). The anterior (front) surface of these tissues is the peritoneum, while the posterior (rear) surface is the transversalis fascia.

The superior pole of the right kidney is adjacent to the liver. For the left kidney, it's next to the spleen. Both, therefore, move down upon inhalation.

In adult males, the kidney weighs between 125 and 170 grams. In females the weight of the kidney is between 115 and 155 grams. A Danish study measured the median renal length to be 11.2 cm (4.4 in) on the left side and 10.9 cm (4.3 in) on the right side in adults. Median renal volumes were 146 cm³ on the left and 134 cm³ on the right.

The substance, or parenchyma, of the kidney is divided into two major structures: the outer renal cortex and the inner renal medulla. Grossly, these structures take the shape of eight to 18 cone-shaped renal lobes, each containing renal cortex surrounding a portion of medulla called a renal pyramid (of Malpighi). Between the renal pyramids are projections of cortex called renal columns (or Bertin columns). Nephrons, the urine-producing functional structures of the kidney, span the cortex and medulla. The initial filtering portion of a nephron is the renal corpuscle which is located in the cortex. This is followed by a renal tubule that passes from the cortex deep into the medullary pyramids. Part of the renal cortex, a medullary ray is a collection of renal tubules that drain into a single collecting duct.

The tip, or papilla, of each pyramid empties urine into a minor calyx; minor calyces empty into major calyces, and major calyces empty into the renal pelvis. This becomes the ureter. At the hilum, the ureter and renal vein exit the kidney and the renal artery enters. Hilar fat and lymphatic tissue with lymph nodes surrounds these structures. The hilar fat is contiguous with a fat-filled cavity called the renal sinus. The renal sinus collectively contains the renal pelvis and calyces and separates these structures from the renal medullary tissue.

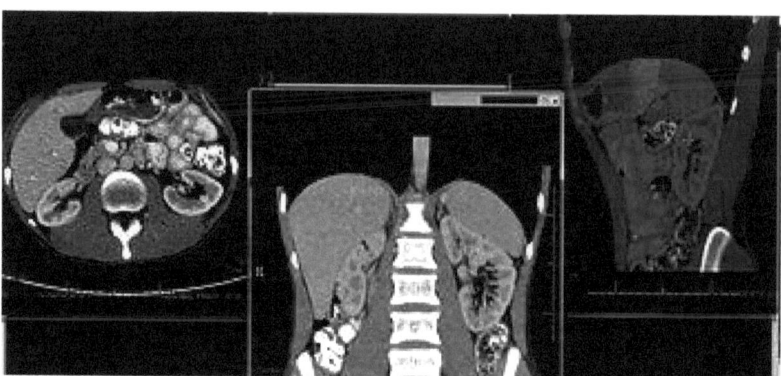

3D-rendered computed tomography, showing renal arteries and veins. The renal circulation supplies the blood to the kidneys via the renal arteries, left and right, which branch directly from the abdominal aorta. Despite their relatively small size, the kidneys receive approximately 20% of the cardiac output.

Each renal artery branches into segmental arteries, dividing further into interlobar arteries, which penetrate the renal capsule and extend through the renal columns between the renal pyramids. The interlobar arteries then supply blood to the arcuate arteries that run through the boundary of the cortex and the medulla. Each arcuate artery supplies several interlobular arteries that feed into the afferent arterioles that supply the glomeruli.

The medullary interstitium is the functional space in the kidney beneath the individual filters (glomeruli), which are rich in blood vessels. The interstitium absorbs fluid recovered from urine. Various conditions can lead to scarring and congestion of this area, which can cause kidney dysfunction and failure.

After filtration occurs, the blood moves through a small network of venules that converge into interlobular veins. As with the arteriole distribution, the veins follow the same pattern: the interlobular provide blood to the arcuate veins then back to the interlobar veins, which come to form the renal vein exiting the kidney for transfusion for blood.

Renal histology studies the microscopic structure of the kidney. Distinct cell types include:

- *Kidney glomerulus parietal cell*
- *Kidney glomerulus podocyte*
- *Kidney proximal tubule brush border cell*
- *Loop of Henle thin segment cell*
- *Thick ascending limb cell*

- *Kidney distal tubule cell*
- *Collecting duct principal cell*
- *Collecting duct intercalated cell*
- *Interstitial kidney cells*

The renal artery enters into the kidney at the level of the first lumbar vertebra just below the superior mesenteric artery. As it enters the kidney, it divides into branches: first the segmental artery, which divides into 2 or 3 lobar arteries, then further divides into interlobar arteries, which further divide into the arcuate artery, which leads into the interlobular artery, which form afferent arterioles. The afferent arterioles form the glomerulus (network of capillaries enclosed in Bowman's capsule). From here, efferent arterioles leaves the glomerulus and divide into peritubular capillaries, which drain into the interlobular veins and then into arcuate vein and then into interlobar vein, which runs into lobar vein, which opens into the segmental vein and which drains into the renal vein, and then from it blood moves into the inferior vena cava.

The kidney participates in whole-body homeostasis, regulating acid-base balance, electrolyte concentrations, extracellular fluid volume, and blood pressure. The kidney accomplishes these homeostatic functions both independently and in concert with other organs, particularly those of the endocrine system. Various endocrine hormones coordinate these endocrine functions; these include renin, angiotensin II, aldosterone, antidiuretic hormone, and atrial natriuretic peptide, among others.

Many of the kidney's functions are accomplished by relatively simple mechanisms of filtration, reabsorption, and secretion, which take place in the nephron. Filtration, which takes place at the renal corpuscle, is the process by which cells and large proteins are filtered from the blood to make an ultrafiltrate that eventually becomes urine. The kidney generates 180 liters of filtrate a day, while reabsorbing a large percentage, allowing for the generation of only approximately 2 liters of urine. Reabsorption is the transport of molecules from this ultrafiltrate and into the blood. Secretion is the reverse process, in which molecules are transported in the opposite direction, from the blood into the urine.

The kidneys excrete a variety of waste products produced by metabolism into the urine. These include the nitrogenous wastes urea, from protein catabolism, and uric acid, from nucleic acid metabolism. The ability of mammals and some birds to concentrate wastes into a volume of urine much smaller than the volume of blood from which the wastes were extracted is dependent on an elaborate countercurrent multiplication mechanism. This requires several independent nephron characteristics to operate: a tight hairpin configuration of the tubules, water and ion permeability in the descending limb of the loop, water impermeability in the ascending loop, and active ion transport out of most of the ascending limb. In addition, passive countercurrent exchange by the vessels carrying the blood supply to the nephron is essential for enabling this function.

Glucose at normal plasma levels is completely reabsorbed in the proximal tubule. The mechanism for this is the Na+/glucose cotransporter. A plasma level of 350 mg/dL will fully saturate the transporters and glucose will be lost in the urine. A plasma glucose level of approximately 160 is sufficient to allow glucosuria, which is an important clinical clue to diabetes mellitus.

Amino acids are reabsorbed by sodium dependent transporters in the proximal tubule. Hartnup disease is a deficiency of the tryptophan amino acid transporter, which results in pellagra.

Pregnancy reduces the reabsorption of glucose and amino acids.

Two organ systems, the kidneys and lungs, maintain acid-base homeostasis, which is the maintenance of pH around a relatively stable value. The lungs contribute to acid-base homeostasis by regulating carbon dioxide ($CO_2$) concentration. The kidneys have two very important roles in maintaining the acid-base balance: to reabsorb and regenerate bicarbonate from urine, and to excrete hydrogen ions and fixed acids (anions of acids) into urine.

Any significant rise in plasma osmolality is detected by the hypothalamus, which communicates directly with the posterior pituitary gland. An increase in osmolality causes the gland to secrete antidiuretic hormone (ADH), resulting in water reabsorption by the kidney and an increase in urine concentration. The two factors work together to return the plasma osmolality to its normal levels.

ADH binds to principal cells in the collecting duct that translocate aquaporins to the membrane, allowing water to leave the normally impermeable membrane and be reabsorbed into the body by the vasa recta, thus increasing the plasma volume of the body.

There are two systems that create a hyperosmotic medulla and thus increase the body plasma volume: Urea recycling and the 'single effect.'

Urea is usually excreted as a waste product from the kidneys. However, when plasma blood volume is low and ADH is released the aquaporins that are opened are also permeable to urea. This allows urea to leave the collecting duct into the medulla creating a hyperosmotic solution that 'attracts' water. Urea can then re-enter the nephron and be excreted or recycled again depending on whether ADH is still present or not.

The 'Single effect' describes the fact that the ascending thick limb of the loop of Henle is not permeable to water but is permeable to NaCl. This allows for a countercurrent exchange system whereby the medulla becomes increasingly concentrated, but at the same time setting up an osmotic gradient for water to follow should the aquaporins of the collecting duct be opened by ADH.

Although the kidney cannot directly sense blood, long-term regulation of blood pressure predominantly depends upon the kidney. This primarily occurs through maintenance of the extracellular fluid compartment, the size of which depends on the plasma sodium concentration. Renin is the first in a series of important chemical messengers that make up the renin-angiotensin system. Changes in renin ultimately alter the output of this system, principally the hormones angiotensin II and aldosterone. Each hormone acts via multiple mechanisms, but both increase the kidney's absorption of sodium chloride, thereby expanding the extracellular fluid compartment and raising blood pressure. When renin levels are elevated, the concentrations of angiotensin II and aldosterone increase, leading to increased sodium chloride reabsorption, expansion of the extracellular fluid compartment, and an increase in blood pressure. Conversely, when renin levels are low, angiotensin II and aldosterone levels decrease, contracting the extracellular fluid compartment, and decreasing blood pressure.

Hormone secretion kidneys secrete a variety of hormones, including erythropoietin, and the enzyme renin. Erythropoietin is released in response to hypoxia (low levels of oxygen at tissue level) in the renal circulation. It stimulates erythropoiesis (production of red blood cells) in the bone marrow. Calcitriol, the activated form of vitamin D, promotes intestinal absorption of calcium and the renal reabsorption of phosphate. Part of the renin–angiotensin–aldosterone system, renin is an enzyme involved in the regulation of aldosterone levels.

## The functional tissues of the heart and the cardiac conduction system

The heart wall is comprised of three layers, the epicardium (outer), myocardium (middle), and endocardium (inner). These tissue layers are highly specialized and perform different functions. During ventricular contraction, the wave of depolarization from the SA and AV nodes moves from within the endocardial wall through the myocardial layer to the epicardial surface of the heart.

*Epicardium*
The outer layer of the heart wall is the epicardium. The epicardium refers to both the outer layer of the heart and the inner layer of the serous visceral pericardium, that is attached to the outer wall of the heart. The epicardium is a thin layer of elastic connective tissue and fat, and serves as an additional layer of protection from trauma or friction for the heart under the pericardium. This layer contains the coronary blood vessels, which oxygenate the tissues of the heart with a blood supply from the coronary arteries.

*Myocardium*
The middle layer of the heart wall is the myocardium—the muscle tissue of the heart and the thickest layer of the heart wall. It is composed of cardiac muscle cells, or cardiomyocytes. Cardiomyocytes are specialized muscle cells that contract like other muscle cells, but differ in shape. Compared to skeletal muscle cells, cardiac muscle cells are shorter and have fewer nuclei. Cardiac muscle tissue is also striated (forming protein bands) and contains tubules and gap junctions, unlike skeletal muscle tissue. Due to their continuous rhythmic contraction, cardiomyocytes require a dedicated blood supply to deliver oxygen and nutrients and remove waste products, such as carbon dioxide, from the cardiac muscle tissue. This blood supply is provided by the coronary arteries.

*Endocardium*

The inner layer of the heart wall is the endocardium, composed of endothelial cells which provide a smooth, elastic, non-adherent surface for blood collection and pumping, and may regulate metabolic waste removal from heart tissues. It is believed that the endocardium acts as a barrier between the blood and the heart muscle, thus controlling the composition of the extracellular fluid in which the cardiomyocytes bathe; this in turn can affect the contractility of the heart. This tissue also covers the valves of the heart, and is histologically continuous with the vascular endothelium of the major blood vessels entering and leaving the heart. The Purkinje fibers are located just beneath the endocardium and send nervous impulses from the SA and AV nodes outside of the heart into the myocardial tissues. The endocardium can be infected, in a serious inflammatory condition called infective endocarditis. Many other problems can occur with the endocardium, which way damage the valves and impair the normal flow of blood through the heart.

Cardiac muscle tissue is an extremely specialized form of muscle tissue that has evolved to pump blood throughout the body. In fact, cardiac muscle is only found in the heart and makes up the bulk of the heart's mass. The heart beats powerfully and continuously throughout an entire lifetime without any rest, so cardiac muscle has evolved to have incredibly high contractile strength and endurance. And because the heart maintains its own rhythm, cardiac muscle has developed the ability to quickly spread electrochemical signals so that all of the cells in the heart can contract together as a team. Cardiac muscle tissue is made up of many interlocking cardiac muscle cells, or fibers, that give the tissue its properties. Each cardiac muscle fiber contains a single nucleus and is striated, or striped, because it appears to have light and dark bands when seen through a microscope. The dark bands represent areas of thick protein filaments made of myosin proteins that block light passing through the cell and appear dark. Between the dark bands are thin filaments made of actin protein that allow light to pass through and appear light. When the muscle fibers contract, myosin pulls the actin filaments together like an accordion to shrink the muscle cell and make it contract. While each cell is not very strong by itself, millions of cardiac muscle cells working together are easily able to pump all of the blood in the body through the heart in less than a minute.

Cardiac muscle cells have a branched shape so that each cell is in contact with three of four other cardiac muscle cells. Together all of the cardiac muscle cells in the heart form a giant network connected end to end. At the ends of each cell is a region of overlapping, finger-like extensions of the cell membrane known as intercalated disks. The intercalated disks form tight junctions between the cells so that they cannot separate under the strain of pumping blood and so that electrochemical signals can be passed quickly from cells to cell. The passage of signals from cell to cell allows cardiac muscle tissue to contract very quickly in a wave-like pattern to effectively pump blood throughout the body.

Another feature that is unique to cardiac muscle tissue is autorhythmicity. Cardiac muscle tissue is able to set its own contraction rhythm due to the presence of pacemaker cells that stimulate the other cardiac muscle cells. The pacemaker cells normally receive inputs from the nervous system to increase or decrease the heart rate depending on the body's needs. However, in the absence of nervous system stimulation, the pacemaker cells can produce a regular heart rhythm.

## The components and function of blood

Blood is a constantly circulating fluid providing the body with nutrition, oxygen, and waste removal. Blood is mostly liquid, with numerous cells and proteins suspended in it, making blood "thicker" than pure water. The average person has about 5 liters (more than a gallon) of blood. A liquid called plasma makes up about half of the content of blood. Plasma contains proteins that help blood to clot, transport substances through the blood, and perform other functions. Blood plasma also contains glucose and other dissolved nutrients.

About half of blood volume is composed of blood cells:

- *Red blood cells, which carry oxygen to the tissues*
- *White blood cells, which fight infections*
- *Platelets, smaller cells that help blood to clot*

Blood is conducted through blood vessels (arteries and veins). Blood is prevented from clotting in the blood vessels by their smoothness, and the finely tuned balance of clotting factors.

Blood Conditions:

*Hemorrhage (bleeding):* Blood leaking out of blood vessels may be obvious, as from a wound penetrating the skin. Internal bleeding (such as into the intestines, or after a car accident) may not be immediately apparent.

*Hematoma:* A collection of blood inside the body tissues. Internal bleeding often causes a hematoma.

*Leukemia:* A form of blood cancer, in which white blood cells multiply abnormally and circulate through the blood. The excessive large numbers of white cells deposit in the body's tissues, causing damage.

*Multiple myeloma:* A form of blood cancer of plasma cells similar to leukemia. Anemia, kidney failure and high blood calcium levels are common in multiple myeloma.

*Lymphoma:* A form of blood cancer, in which white blood cells multiply abnormally inside lymph nodes and other tissues. The enlarging tissues, and disruption of blood's functions, can eventually cause organ failure.

*Anemia:* An abnormally low number of red blood cells in the blood. Fatigue and breathlessness can result, although anemia often causes no noticeable symptoms.

*Hemolytic anemia:* Anemia caused by rapid bursting of large numbers of red blood cells (hemolysis). An immune system malfunction is one cause.

*Hemochromatosis:* A disorder causing excessive levels of iron in the blood. The iron deposits in the liver, pancreas and other organs, causing liver problems and diabetes.

*Sickle cell disease:* A genetic condition in which red blood cells periodically lose their proper shape (appearing like sickles, rather than discs). The deformed blood cells deposit in tissues, causing pain and organ damage.

*Bacteremia:* Bacterial infection of the blood. Blood infections are serious, and often require hospitalization and continuous antibiotic infusion into the veins.

*Malaria:* Infection of red blood cells by Plasmodium, a parasite transmitted by mosquitos. Malaria causes episodic fevers, chills, and potentially organ damage.

*Thrombocytopenia:* Abnormally low numbers of platelets in the blood. Severe thrombocytopenia may lead to bleeding.

*Leukopenia:* Abnormally low numbers of white blood cells in the blood. Leukopenia can result in difficulty fighting infections.

*Disseminated intravascular coagulation (DIC):* An uncontrolled process of simultaneous bleeding and clotting in very small blood vessels. DIC usually results from severe infections or cancer.

*Hemophilia:* An inherited (genetic) deficiency of certain blood clotting proteins. Frequent or uncontrolled bleeding can result from hemophilia.

*Hypercoaguable state:* Numerous conditions can result in the blood being prone to clotting. A heart attack, stroke, or blood clots in the legs or lungs can result.

*Polycythemia:* Abnormally high numbers of red blood cells in the blood. Polycythemia can result from low blood oxygen levels, or may occur as a cancer-like condition.

*Deep venous thrombosis (DVT):* A blood clot in a deep vein, usually in the leg. DVTs are dangerous because they may become dislodged and travel to the lungs, causing a pulmonary embolism (PE).

*Myocardial infarction (MI):* Commonly called a heart attack, a myocardial infarction occurs when a sudden blood clot develops in one of the coronary arteries, which supply blood to the heart.

## The cardiac cycle with diagram

The cardiac cycle refers to a complete heartbeat from its generation to the beginning of the next beat, and so includes the diastole, the systole, and the intervening pause. The frequency of the cardiac cycle is described by the heart rate, which is typically expressed as beats per minute. Each beat of the heart involves five major stages. The first two stages, often considered together as the "ventricular filling" stage, involve the movement of blood from the atria into the ventricles. The next three stages involve the movement of blood from the ventricles to the pulmonary artery (in the case of the right ventricle) and the aorta (in the case of the left ventricle).

The first stage, "diastole," is when the semilunar valves (the pulmonary valve and the aortic valve) close, the atrioventricular (AV) valves (the mitral valve and the tricuspid valve) open, and the whole heart is relaxed. The second stage, "atrial systole," is when the atrium contracts, and blood flows from atrium to the ventricle. The third stage, "isovolumic contraction" is when the ventricles begin to contract, the AV and semilunar valves close, and there is no change in volume. The fourth stage, "ventricular ejection," is when the ventricles are contracting and emptying, and the semilunar valves are open. During the fifth stage, "isovolumic relaxation time", pressure decreases, no blood enters the ventricles, the ventricles stop contracting and begin to relax, and the semilunar valves close due to the pressure of blood in the aorta.

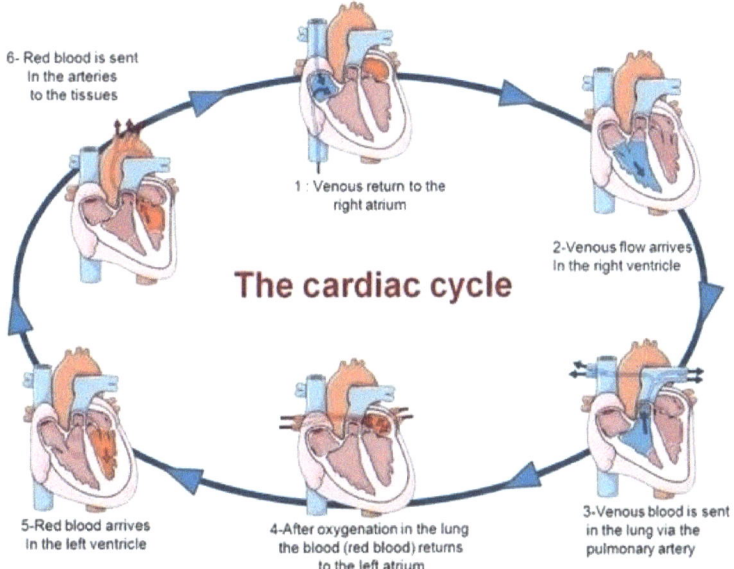

Throughout the cardiac cycle, blood pressure increases and decreases. The cardiac cycle is coordinated by a series of electrical impulses that are produced by specialised pacemaker cells found within the sinoatrial node and the atrioventricular node. The cardiac muscle is composed of myocytes which initiate their own contraction without the help of external nerves (with the exception of modifying the heart rate due to metabolic demand). Under normal circumstances, each cycle takes 0.6666 seconds. The heart is a four-chambered organ consisting of right and left halves. The upper two chambers, the left and right atria, are entry-points into the heart, while the lower two chambers, the left and right

[95]

ventricles, are responsible for contractions that send the blood through the circulation. The circulation is split into the pulmonary and systemic circulation. The role of the right ventricle is to pump deoxygenated blood to the lungs through the pulmonary trunk and pulmonary arteries. The role of the left ventricle is to pump newly oxygenated blood to the body through the aorta.

Cardiac muscle has automaticity, which means that it is self-exciting. The muscle contractions are myogenic, or generated by the muscle cell itself. This is in contrast with skeletal muscle, which requires nervous stimuli (either conscious or reflex) for excitation. The heart's rhythmic contractions occur spontaneously, although the rate of contraction can be changed by nervous or hormonal influences. For example, the sympathetic nerve accelerates heart rate and the vagus nerve decelerates the heart rate.

The rhythmic sequence of contractions (sinus rhythm), is coordinated by the sinoatrial (SA) and atrioventricular (AV) nodes. The sinoatrial node, often known as the cardiac pacemaker, is located in the upper wall of the right atrium and is responsible for the wave of electrical stimulation that initiates atrial contraction by creating an action potential. Once the wave reaches the AV node, situated in the lower right atrium, it is delayed there before being conducted through the bundles of His and back up the Purkinje fibers, leading to a contraction of the ventricles. The delay at the AV node allows enough time for all of the blood in the atria to fill their respective ventricles. In the event of severe pathology, the AV node can also act as a pacemaker; this is usually not the case because its rate of spontaneous firing is considerably lower than that of the SA node and hence it is overridden.

## The concepts of spermatogenesis and oogenesis

Both spermatogenesis and oogenesis are commonly referred to as gametogenesis. Gametogenesis is the series of mitotic and meiotic divisions occurring in the gonads, to form gametes. The gamete production is very much different among males and females; thus the production of gametes in males is called spermatogenesis, whereas that of females is called oogenesis. Even though there are meiosis and mitosis, both are present during gametogenesis; the actual formation of gametes begins with the meiosis.

*Spermatogenesis*

Formation of spermatids (sperm cells) in male testes is referred to as spermatogenesis. The process starts from spermatogonium, which are genetically diploid. Spermatogonia produce primary spermatocyte (diploid) through mitosis. The resulting primary spermatocyte undergoes meiosis I to produce two identical haploid cells called secondary spermatocytes. Each spermatocyte again divides through meiosis II, to form two haploid daughter cells called spermatids. Thus, one primary spermatocyte produces four identical haploid spermatids. It takes about 6 weeks to differentiate spermatid into mature spermatozoa.

Oogenesis is the formation of eggs in females. Usually, the initial stages of oogenesis start during early embryonic stages and completes after puberty. The production of ovum has a cyclic pattern and, usually occurs once in a month. Oogenesis starts from the diploid oogonium in the ovary. Primary oocytes are produced from oogonia by mitosis during the early embryonic developmental stages. After the puberty, these primary oocytes start to convert to secondary oocytes, which are haploid, during the meiosis I. Then during the meiosis II, secondary oocyte converts to ovum, which is also haploid. During both meiosis I and II, the cytoplasm divides unequally, producing two unequal sized cells. The larger cell becomes the ovum while the smaller one becomes polar body. The secondary oocyte is released from the ovary at ovulation.

Spermatogenesis is the production of sperm cells in males, whereas oogenesis is the production of ovum in females.

In vertebrates, Spermatogenesis occurs in male testes, whereas oogenesis occurs in female ovary.

Spermatogenesis starts from a primary spermatocyte while oogenesis starts from a primary oocyte.

Spermatogenesis results four functional spermatozoa from a primary spermatocyte. In contrast, oogenesis results a single ovum and three polar bodies from a primary oocyte.

In spermatogenesis, cytokinesis results in two equal sized cells while, in oogenesis, it results in two highly unequal cells.

- Sperm cell does not contain any food, unlike the ovum (egg).
- Sperm cells are much smaller than egg.
- Sperm cells are motile, whereas ovum is immotile.
- Spermatogenesis is completed while it's inside the testis. In contrast, secondary maturation division in oogenesis occurs outside the ovary (it occurs in the oviduct).
- Spermatogenesis begins at puberty, whereas oogenesis begins even before the birth, during the embryonic developmental stages.
- Spermatogenesis results billions of sperm cells at one, whereas oogenesis result only one ovum per month.
- Spermatogenesis involves a short growth phase while oogenesis involves a long one.
- Unlike the spermatogenesis, the process of oogenesis depends on the amount of York stored in the ova in different groups of vertebrates.
- Spermatogenesis occurs continuously after the puberty, whereas oogenesis occurs in a cyclic pattern.

## Classification of tissues with examples

There are several major types of tissues. The most common types are epithelial, connective, muscle, and nervous tissues. Tissues make up organs. An organ is a structure performing a particular function. An organ is composed of several different tissues.

Epithelial tissue is tissue that covers surfaces and lines cavities. Here, it may protect, absorb, and/or secrete. Epithelial tissue covers the outer surface of the body. It lines the intestines, the lungs, and other hollow organs.

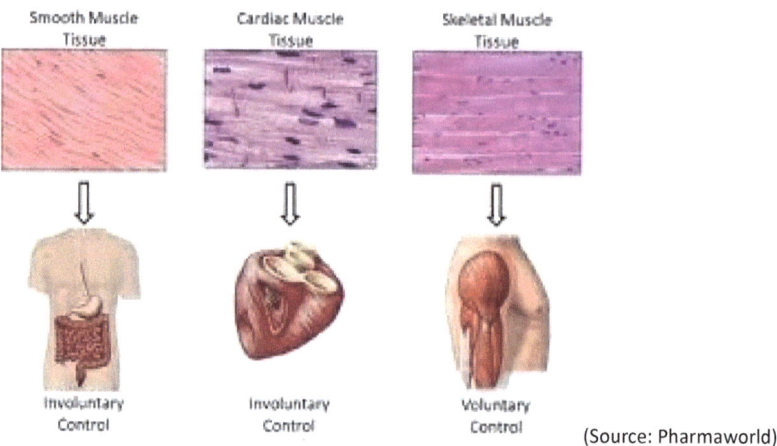

(Source: Pharmaworld)

*Types of epithelial cells (by shape)*
The three basic shapes are squamous (flat), cuboidal (cubes), and columnar (columns).

*Types of epithelial tissues*
a. Layers. In epithelial tissues, the cells are in single or multiple layers. If there is only one layer, the tissue is called a simple epithelium. If there is more than one layer, the tissue is called a stratified epithelium. Epithelial tissues are named by the number of layers and the type of cell in its outermost layer. For example, if there are several layers and if the outermost layer consists of squamous (flat) cells, then the tissue is called a stratified squamous epithelium.

(1) A simple squamous epithelium called endothelium lines the heart and blood vessels.

(2) As serous membranes, simple squamous epithelial tissue lines the cavities of the abdomen (peritoneal lining) and the chest (pleural lining). Serous membranes are membranes which secrete a lubricating fluid.

(3) Epithelial tissue forms the secretory part of glands and also parts of the various sense organs.

According to its location, epithelial tissue has different functions. As the skin, epithelial tissue protects the tissues beneath. In the small intestines, the epithelial tissue absorbs. In the lungs, epithelial tissue is a membrane through which the gases pass easily. In the glands, epithelial tissue secretes.

*Definition of connective tissues*

Connective tissue is tissue that supports other tissues, holds tissues together, or fills spaces. Among and outside the cells of the connective tissues, there is a material called matrix. The matrix is manufactured by the connective tissue cells. Each type of connective tissue has its own particular type of matrix.

*Types of connective tissue*

There are several major types of connective tissue (CT). These include fibrous CT (FCT), cartilage CT, bone CT, and fat CT. Blood is sometimes considered an additional type of CT.

*Fibrous connective tissue (FCT)*

a. Fibroblasts. The characteristic cells of FCT are fibroblasts. Fibroblasts are able
to form elongated fibers.
b. Matrix. These fibers make up the matrix of FCT.
c. Fibers. The fibers are either white or yellow.
(1) White fibers are made from a protein called collagen. White fibers tend to
have a fixed length. White fibers are not very easily stretched.
(2) Yellow fibers are made from a protein called elastin. Yellow fibers are elastic.
They can be stretched and then they can snap back (like a rubber band).
d. Types of FCT. The types of FCT are recognized by the arrangement of their
fibers. These types include:
(1) Loose areolar FCT. Loose areolar FCT has an open irregular arrangement of its fibers. Loose areolar FCT is found widely throughout the body. An example is the superficial fascia (subcutaneous layer). The superficial fascia is the connective tissue which lies beneath the skin. Loose areolar FCT is the filling substance around most organs and tissues of the body.
(2) Dense FCT. The fibers of dense FCT are closely packed and parallel. There are no significant spaces between the fibers. Examples of dense FCT are ligaments and tendons. A ligament is a band of dense FCT that holds the bones together at a joint. A tendon attaches a muscle to a bone.

*Cartilage connective tissue*

a. Cartilage Cells. Cartilage cells are also called chondroblasts. Cartilage cells are clustered in microscopic pockets within the cartilage matrix. The cartilage cells produce the material of the matrix.
b. Matrix. The matrix produced by the cartilage cells appears homogeneous (the same throughout). The matrix also appears amorphous (shapeless).
c. Types of Cartilage CT.
(1) Hyaline cartilage CT. Hyaline cartilage CT appears homogeneous and clear. This type of cartilage helps to cover bone surfaces at joints. Hyaline cartilage is found as incomplete rings which keep the trachea (windpipe) open.
(2) Fibrous cartilage CT. Fibrous cartilage CT includes dense masses of fibers (of FCT). It is more rigid than hyaline cartilage. The auricle of the external ear is stiffened with fibrous cartilage.
(3) Calcified cartilage CT. Calcified cartilage CT is cartilage that has been stiffened

by the addition of calcium salts. This is not the same as bone tissue. An example is the cartilages of the larynx (the voice box) which become calcified with age.

*Bone connective tissue*
a. Osteoblasts/Osteoclasts. Osteoblasts are cells that make and repair bone. Osteoclasts are cells which tear down and remove bone. Bone is continually being remodeled as a person lives. Remodeling is in direct response to the stresses placed on the bone.
b. Types of Bone Tissues. There are two major types of bone tissue. One is compact bone CT, which is dense. The other is cancellous bone CT, which is spongy. Compact bone CT forms the hard outer layers of bones as organs. Cancellous bone CT forms the inner, lighter portion of bones.

*Fat connective tissue*
a. Fat Cells. A large fraction of the volume of a fat cell is occupied by a droplet of fat. This droplet has its own membrane, in addition to the outer membrane of the cell. The remaining components of the fat cell, including the nucleus, are found in an outer layer of cytoplasm surrounding the droplet of fat.
b. Matrix. Fat connective tissue has a matrix of lipid (oil or fat). There may be yellow fat CT or brown fat CT.
c. Functions. Fat CT acts as a packing material among the organs, nerves, and vessels. Fat CT also helps to insulate the body from both heat and cold. Some fat CT serves as a high-energy storage area.

*Blood "connective tissue"*
Some experts consider blood to be a type of connective tissue.

*Definition of muscle tissue*
There are muscle tissues and there are organs called muscles. Muscles are made up of muscle tissues. Muscle tissues and the muscles they make up are specialized to contract. Because of their ability to shorten (contract), muscles are able to
produce motion.

*Types of muscle tissues*
a. Skeletal Muscle Tissue. The cells (muscle fibers) of skeletal muscle tissue are long and cylindrical and have numerous nuclei. The arrangement of the cellular contents is very specific and results in a striated appearance when viewed with the microscope. This type of muscle tissue is found mainly in the skeletal muscles.
b. Cardiac Muscle Tissue. The cells (muscle fibers) of cardiac muscle tissue are short, branched, contain one nucleus, and are striated. This tissue makes up the myocardium (wall) of the heart.
c. Smooth Muscle Tissue. The cells (muscle fibers) of smooth muscle tissue are spindle-shaped, contain one nucleus, and are not striated. Smooth muscle tissue
is generally found in the walls of hollow organs such as the organs of the digestive and respiratory systems, the blood vessels, the ureters, urinary bladder, urethra, and reproductive ducts.

*Definition of nervous tissue*

Nervous tissue is a collection of cells that respond to stimuli and transmit information.

*Nervous tissue cells*

a. A neuron, or nerve cell, is the cell of the nervous tissue that actually picks up and transmits a signal from one part of the body to another. A synapse is the point at which a signal passes from one neuron to the next.

b. The neuroglia (also known as glia) is made up of the supporting cells of the nervous system (glial cells).

Example: The skin is the largest organ of the body, with a total area of about 20 square feet. The skin protects us from microbes and the elements, helps regulate body temperature, and permits the sensations of touch, heat, and cold.

Skin has three layers: The epidermis, the outermost layer of skin, provides a waterproof barrier and creates our skin tone. The dermis, beneath the epidermis, contains tough connective tissue, hair follicles, and sweat glands. The deeper subcutaneous tissue (hypodermis) is made of fat and connective tissue. The skin's colour is created by special cells called melanocytes, which produce the pigment melanin. Melanocytes are located in the epidermis.

## 8. Pathology

### Pathology and the knowledge of medicine-Justification

Pathology (from the Greek roots of pathos (πάθος), meaning "experience" or "suffering", and -logia (-λογία), "study of") is a significant component of the causal study of disease and a major field in modern medicine and diagnosis. The term pathology itself may be used broadly to refer to the study of disease in general, incorporating a wide range of bioscience research fields and medical practices (including plant pathology and veterinary pathology), or more narrowly to describe work within the contemporary medical field of "general pathology," which includes a number of distinct but inter-related medical specialties that diagnose disease—mostly through analysis of tissue, cell, and body fluid samples. Used as a count noun, "a pathology" (plural, "pathologies") can also refer to the predicted or actual progression of particular diseases (as in the statement "the many different forms of cancer have diverse pathologies"), and the affix path is sometimes used to indicate a state of disease in cases of both physical ailment (as in cardiomyopathy) and psychological conditions (such as psychopathy). Similarly, a pathological condition is one caused by disease, rather than occurring physiologically.

## Immunity and its classification with examples

Immunity or Immunopathology is a branch of clinical pathology that deals with an organism's immune response to a certain disease. When a foreign antigen enters the body, there is either an antigen specific or nonspecific response to it. These responses are the immune system fighting off the foreign antigens, whether they are deadly or not. Immunopathology could refer to how the foreign antigens cause the immune system to have a response or problems that can arise from an organism's own immune response on itself. There are certain problems or faults in the immune system that can lead to more serious illness or disease. These diseases can come from one of the following problems. The first would be Hypersensitivity reactions, where there would be a stronger immune response than normal. There are four different types (type one, two, three and four), all with varying types and degrees of an immune response. The problems that arise from each type vary from small allergic reactions to more serious illnesses such as tuberculosis or arthritis.

The second kind of complication in the immune system is Autoimmunity, where the immune system would attack itself rather than the antigen. Inflammation is a prime example of autoimmunity, as the immune cells used are self-reactive. A few examples of autoimmune diseases are Type 1 diabetes, Addison's disease and Celiac disease. The third and final type of complication with the immune system is Immunodeficiency, where the immune system lacks the ability to fight off a certain disease. The immune system's ability to combat it is either hindered or completely absent. The two types are Primary Immunodeficiency, where the immune system is either missing a key component or does not function properly, and Secondary Immunodeficiency, where disease is obtained from an outside source, like radiation or heat, and therefore cannot function properly. Diseases that can cause immunodeficiency include HIV, AIDS and leukemia. In all vertebrates, there are two different kinds of immune responses: Innate and Adaptive immunity. Innate immunity is used to fight off non-changing antigens and is therefore considered nonspecific. It is usually a more immediate response than the adaptive immune system, usually responding within minutes to hours.[18] It is composed of physical blockades such as the skin, but also contains nonspecific immune cells such as dendritic cells, macrophages, T Cells, and basophils. The second for of immunity is Adaptive immunity. This form of immunity requires recognition of the foreign antigen before a response is produced. Once the antigen is recognized, a specific response is produced in order to destroy the specific antigen. Because of this idea, adaptive immunity is considered to be specific immunity.

A key part of adaptive immunity that separates it from innate is the use of memory to combat the antigen in the future. When the antigen is originally introduced, the organism does not have any receptors for the antigen so it must generate them from the first time the antigen is present. The immune system then builds a memory of that antigen, which enables it to recognize the antigen quicker in the future and be able to combat it quicker and more efficiently. The more the system is exposed to the antigen, the quicker it will build up its responsiveness

## Pathology: What are its branches? Why should we study it in medical science?

The modern practice of pathology is divided into a number of subdisciplines within the discrete but deeply interconnected aims of biological research and medical practice. Biomedical research into disease incorporates the work of vast variety of life science specialists, whereas, in most parts of the world, to be licensed to practice pathology as medical specialty, one has to complete medical school and secure a license to practice medicine. Structurally, the study of disease is divided into many different fields that study or diagnose markers for disease using methods and technologies particular to specific scales, organs, and tissue types. The information in this section mostly concerns pathology as it regards common medical practice in these systems, but each of these specialties is also the subject of voluminous pathology research as regards the disease pathways of specific pathogens and disorders that affect the tissues of these discrete organs or structures. Pathology contains the following subdisciplines:

Anatomical pathology

- *Cytopathology*
- *Dermatopathology*
- *Forensic pathology*
- *Histopathology*
- *Neuropathology*
- *Pulmonary pathology*
- *Renal pathology*
- *Surgical pathology*

Clinical pathology

- Hematopathology
- Immunopathology
- Radiation Pathology

Molecular pathology

Oral and maxillofacial pathology

## Pyogenic Organisms: How to proceed to isolate and diagnose pulmonary tuberculosis

Pus is an exudate, typically white-yellow, yellow, or yellow-brown, formed at the site of inflammation during bacterial or fungal infection. An accumulation of pus in an enclosed tissue space is known as an abscess, whereas a visible collection of pus within or beneath the epidermis is known as a pustule, pimple, or spot.

Pus consists of a thin, protein-rich fluid, known as liquor puris, and dead leukocytes from the body's immune response (mostly neutrophils)[citation needed]. During infection, macrophages release cytokines which trigger neutrophils to seek the site of infection by chemotaxis. There, the neutrophils release granules which destroy the bacteria. The bacteria resist the immune response by releasing toxins called leukocidins. As the neutrophils die off from toxins and old age, they are destroyed by macrophages, forming the viscous pus. Bacteria that cause pus are called pyogenic.

Although pus is normally of a whitish-yellow hue, changes in the color can be observed under certain circumstances. Pus is sometimes green because of the presence of myeloperoxidase, an intensely green antibacterial protein produced by some types of white blood cells. Green, foul-smelling pus is found in certain infections of Pseudomonas aeruginosa. The greenish color is a result of the bacterial pigment pyocyanin that it produces. Amoebic abscesses of the liver produce brownish pus, which is described as looking like "anchovy paste". Pus can also have a foul odor, particularly pus from anaerobic infections. In almost all cases when there is a collection of pus in the body, the clinician will try to create an opening to drain it. This principle has been distilled into the famous Latin aphorism "Ubi pus, ibi evacua" ("Where there is pus, evacuate it").

Pyogenic bacteria

A great many species of bacteria may be involved in the production of pus. The most commonly found include:

- *Staphylococcus aureus*
- *Staphylococcus epidermidis*
- *Streptococcus pyogenes*
- *Escherichia coli (Bacillus coli communis)*
- *Streptococcus pneumoniae (Fraenkel's pneumococcus)*
- *Klebsiella pneumoniae (Friedländer's bacillus)*
- *Salmonella typhi (Bacillus typhosus)*
- *Pseudomonas aeruginosa*
- *Neisseria gonorrhoeae*
- *Actinomyces*
- *Burkholderia mallei (Glanders bacillus)*
- *Mycobacterium tuberculosis (tubercle bacillus)*
- *Staphylococcus aureus bacteria is the most common cause of boils.*

Some disease processes caused by pyogenic infections are impetigo, osteomyelitis, septic arthritis, and necrotizing fasciitis.

If a tuberculosis infection does become active, it most commonly involves the lungs (in about 90% of cases). Symptoms may include chest pain and a prolonged cough producing sputum. About 25% of people may not have any symptoms (i.e. they remain "asymptomatic"). Occasionally, people may cough up blood in small amounts, and in very rare cases, the infection may erode into the pulmonary artery or a Rasmussen's aneurysm, resulting in massive bleeding. Tuberculosis may become a chronic illness and cause extensive scarring in the upper lobes of the lungs. The upper lung lobes are more frequently affected by tuberculosis than the lower ones. The reason for this difference is not clear. It may be due either to better air flow, or to poor lymph drainage within the upper lungs. Treatment of TB uses antibiotics to kill the bacteria. Effective TB treatment is difficult, due to the unusual structure and chemical composition of the mycobacterial cell wall, which hinders the entry of drugs and makes many antibiotics ineffective. The two antibiotics most commonly used are isoniazid and rifampicin, and treatments can be prolonged, taking several months. Latent TB treatment usually employs a single antibiotic, while active TB disease is best treated with combinations of several antibiotics to reduce the risk of the bacteria developing antibiotic resistance.People with latent infections are also treated to prevent them from progressing to active TB disease later in life. Directly observed therapy, i.e., having a health care provider watch the person take their medications, is recommended by the WHO in an effort to reduce the number of people not appropriately taking antibiotics. The evidence to support this practice over people simply taking their medications independently is poor. Methods to remind people of the importance of treatment do, however, appear effective.

## The identification and laboratory diagnosis of enteric fever

Typhoid a form of enteric fever, also known simply as typhoid, is a bacterial infection due to Salmonella typhi that causes symptoms which may vary from mild to severe and usually begin six to thirty days after exposure. Often there is a gradual onset of a high fever over several days. Weakness, abdominal pain, constipation, and headaches also commonly occur. Diarrhea is uncommon and vomiting is not usually severe. Some people develop a skin rash with rose colored spots. In severe cases there may be confusion. Without treatment symptoms may last weeks or months. Other people may carry the bacterium without being affected; however, they are still able to spread the disease to others. Typhoid fever is a type of enteric fever along with paratyphoid fever.

The cause is the bacterium Salmonella typhi, also known as Salmonella enterica serotype typhi, growing in the intestines and blood. Typhoid is spread by eating or drinking food or water contaminated with the feces of an infected person. Risk factors include poor sanitation and poor hygiene. Those who travel to the developing world are also at risk and only humans can be infected. Diagnosis is by either culturing the bacteria or detecting the bacterium's DNA in the blood, stool, or bone marrow. Culturing the bacterium can be difficult. Bone marrow testing is the most accurate. Symptoms are similar to that of many other infectious diseases. Typhus is a different disease. A typhoid vaccine can prevent about 30% to 70% of cases during the first two years. The vaccine may have some effect for up to seven years. It is recommended for those at high risk or people traveling to areas where the disease is common. Other efforts to prevent the disease include providing clean drinking water, better sanitation, and better handwashing. Until it has been confirmed that an individual's infection is cleared, the individual should not prepare food for others. Treatment of disease is with antibiotics such as azithromycin, fluoroquinolones or third generation cephalosporins. Resistance to these antibiotics has been developing, which has made treatment of the disease more difficult.

## Neoplasm and its differences between benign and malignant tumors

Neoplasm is an abnormal growth of tissue and when it also forms a mass is commonly referred to as a tumor. This abnormal growth (neoplasia) usually but not always forms a mass. The World Health Organization (WHO) classifies neoplasms into four main groups: benign neoplasms, in situ neoplasms, malignant neoplasms, and neoplasms of uncertain or unknown behaviour. Malignant neoplasms are also simply known as cancers.
Prior to the abnormal growth of tissue, as neoplasia, cells often undergo an abnormal pattern of growth, such as metaplasia or dysplasia. However, metaplasia or dysplasia does not always progress to neoplasia. A neoplasm can be benign, potentially malignant, or malignant (cancer).

Benign tumors include uterine fibroids and melanocytic nevi (skin moles). They are circumscribed and localized and do not transform into cancer. Potentially-malignant neoplasms include carcinoma in situ. They are localised, do not invade and destroy but in time, may transform into a cancer. Malignant neoplasms are commonly called cancer. They invade and destroy the surrounding tissue, may form metastases and, if untreated or unresponsive to treatment, will prove fatal. Secondary neoplasm refers to any of a class of cancerous tumor that is either a metastatic offshoot of a primary tumor, or an apparently unrelated tumor that increases in frequency following certain cancer treatments such as chemotherapy or radiotherapy. Rarely there can be a metastatic neoplasm with no known site of the primary cancer and this is classed as a cancer of unknown primary origin.

## Koch's postulates, its significances and demerits

Koch's postulates are the following:
The microorganism must be found in abundance in all organisms suffering from the disease, but should not be found in healthy organisms.

The microorganism must be isolated from a diseased organism and grown in pure culture.

The cultured microorganism should cause disease when introduced into a healthy organism.

The microorganism must be reisolated from the inoculated, diseased experimental host and identified as being identical to the original specific causative agent.

However, Koch abandoned the universalist requirement of the first postulate altogether when he discovered asymptomatic carriers of cholera and, later, of typhoid fever. Asymptomatic or subclinical infection carriers are now known to be a common feature of many infectious diseases, especially viruses such as polio, herpes simplex, HIV, and hepatitis C. As a specific example, all doctors and virologists agree that poliovirus causes paralysis in just a few infected subjects, and the success of the polio vaccine in preventing disease supports the conviction that the poliovirus is the causative agent.

The second postulate may also be suspended for certain microorganisms or entities that cannot (at the present time) be grown in pure culture, such as prions responsible for Creutzfeldt–Jakob disease. Viruses also require host cells to grow and reproduce and therefore cannot be grown in pure cultures.

The third postulate specifies "should", not "must", because as Koch himself proved in regard to both tuberculosis and cholera, not all organisms exposed to an infectious agent will acquire the infection. Noninfection may be due to such factors as general health and proper immune functioning; acquired immunity from previous exposure or vaccination; or genetic immunity, as with the resistance to malaria conferred by possessing at least one sickle cell allele. In summary, a body of evidence that satisfies Koch's postulates is sufficient but not necessary to establish causation.

## Necrosis and its aetiology and types

Necrosis is caused by factors external to the cell or tissue, such as infection, toxins, or trauma which result in the unregulated digestion of cell components. In contrast, apoptosis is a naturally occurring programmed and targeted cause of cellular death. While apoptosis often provides beneficial effects to the organism, necrosis is almost always detrimental and can be fatal.

Cellular death due to necrosis does not follow the apoptotic signal transduction pathway, but rather various receptors are activated, and result in the loss of cell membrane integrity and an uncontrolled release of products of cell death into the extracellular space.

This initiates in the surrounding tissue an inflammatory response which prevents nearby phagocytes from locating and eliminating the dead cells by phagocytosis. For this reason, it is often necessary to remove necrotic tissue surgically, a procedure known as debridement. Untreated necrosis results in a build-up of decomposing dead tissue and cell debris at or near the site of the cell death. A classic example is gangrene.

There are six distinctive morphological patterns of necrosis:

a)      Coagulative necrosis is characterized by the formation of a gelatinous (gel-like) substance in dead tissues in which the architecture of the tissue is maintained, and can be observed by light microscopy. Coagulation occurs as a result of protein denaturation, causing albumin to transform into a firm and opaque state. This pattern of necrosis is typically seen in hypoxic (low-oxygen) environments, such as infarction. Coagulative necrosis occurs primarily in tissues such as the kidney, heart and adrenal glands. Severe ischemia most commonly causes necrosis of this form.

b)      Liquefactive necrosis (or colliquative necrosis), in contrast to coagulative necrosis, is characterized by the digestion of dead cells to form a viscous liquid mass. This is typical of bacterial, or sometimes fungal, infections because of their ability to stimulate an inflammatory response. The necrotic liquid mass is frequently creamy yellow due to the presence of dead leukocytes and is commonly known as pus. Hypoxic infarcts in the brain presents as this type of necrosis, because the brain contains little connective tissue but high amounts of digestive enzymes and lipids, and cells therefore can be readily digested by their own enzymes.

c)      Gangrenous necrosis can be considered a type of coagulative necrosis that resembles mummified tissue. It is characteristic of ischemia of lower limb and the gastrointestinal tracts. If superimposed infection of dead tissues occurs, then liquefactive necrosis ensues (wet gangrene).

d)      Caseous necrosis can be considered a combination of coagulative and liquefactive necrosis, typically caused by mycobacteria (e.g. tuberculosis), fungi and some foreign substances. The necrotic tissue appears as white and friable, like clumped cheese. Dead cells disintegrate but are not completely digested, leaving granular particles. Microscopic examination shows amorphous granular debris enclosed within a distinctive inflammatory border. Granuloma has this characteristic.

e)      Fat necrosis is specialized necrosis of fat tissue, resulting from the action of activated lipases on fatty tissues such as the pancreas. In the pancreas it leads to acute pancreatitis, a condition where the pancreatic enzymes leak out into the peritoneal cavity, and liquefy the membrane by splitting the triglyceride esters into fatty acids through fat saponification. Calcium, magnesium or sodium may bind to these lesions to produce a chalky-white substance. The calcium deposits are microscopically distinctive and may be large enough to be visible on radiographic examinations. To the naked eye, calcium deposits appear as gritty white flecks.

f)      Fibrinoid necrosis is a special form of necrosis usually caused by immune-mediated vascular damage. It is marked by complexes of antigen and antibodies, sometimes referred to as "immune complexes" deposited within arterial walls together with fibrin.

## Definition of benign tumors

A benign tumor is a mass of cells (tumor) that lacks the ability to invade neighboring tissue or metastasize. These characteristics are required for a tumor to be defined as cancerous and therefore benign tumors are non-cancerous. Also, benign tumors generally have a slower growth rate than malignant tumors and the tumor cells are usually more differentiated (cells have normal features). Benign tumors are typically surrounded by an outer surface (fibrous sheath of connective tissue) or remain with the epithelium. Common examples of benign tumors include moles and uterine fibroids.

Although benign tumors will not metastasize or locally invade tissues, some types may still produce negative health effects. The growth of benign tumors produces a "mass effect" that can compress tissues and may cause nerve damage, reduction of blood to an area of the body (ischaemia), tissue death (necrosis) and organ damage. The mass effects of tumors are more prominent if the tumor is within an enclosed space such as the cranium, respiratory tract, sinus or inside bones. Tumors of endocrine tissues may overproduce certain hormones, especially when the cells are well differentiated. Examples include thyroid adenomas and adrenocortical adenomas.

Although most benign tumors are not life-threatening, many types of benign tumors have the potential to become cancerous (malignant) through a process known as tumour progression. For this reason and other possible negative health effects, some benign tumors are removed by surgery.

## Definition and classification of shock, the pathogenesis and clinical presentation

Circulatory shock, commonly known as shock, is a life-threatening medical condition of low blood perfusion to tissues resulting in cellular injury and inadequate tissue function. The typical signs of shock are low blood pressure, rapid heart rate, signs of poor end-organ perfusion (i.e.: low urine output, confusion, or loss of consciousness), and weak pulses.

The shock index (SI), defined as heart rate divided by systolic blood pressure, is an accurate diagnostic measure that is more useful than hypotension and tachycardia in isolation. Under normal conditions, a number between 0.5 and 0.8 is typically seen. Should that number increase, so does suspicion of an underlying state of shock. Blood pressure alone may not be a reliable sign for shock, as there are times when a person is in circulatory shock but has a stable blood pressure.

Circulatory shock is not related to the emotional state of shock. Circulatory shock is a life-threatening medical emergency and one of the most common causes of death for critically ill people. Shock can have a variety of effects, all with similar outcomes, but all relate to a problem with the body's circulatory system. For example, shock may lead to hypoxemia (a lack of oxygen in arterial blood) or cardiac and/or respiratory arrest.

One of the key dangers of shock is that it progresses by a positive feedback mechanism. Poor blood supply leads to cellular damage, which results in an inflammatory response to increase blood flow to the affected area. This is normally very useful to match up supply with tissue demand for nutrients. However, if enough tissue causes this, it will deprive vital nutrients from other parts of the body. Additionally, the ability of the circulatory system to meet this increase in demand causes saturation. A major result of which is that other parts of the body begin to respond in a similar way, thus exacerbating the problem. Due to this chain of events, immediate treatment of shock is critical to survival.

www.ingramcontent.com/pod-product-compliance
Lightning Source LLC
Chambersburg PA
CBHW041313180526
45172CB00004B/1083